Achilles Healing

Achilles Tendinitis Relief and Prevention in 4 Easy Phases

Patrick Hafner

Birchbark Publishing

Publisher's Cataloging in Publication

Hafner, Patrick

Achilles Healing: achilles tendinitis relief and prevention in 4 easy phases / Patrick Hafner

p.   cm.

ISBN-13: 978-0-9801724-6-1

1. Achilles injury -- rehabilitation   2. Foot injury -- healing   I. Title

"The natural healing force within each one of us is the greatest force in getting well."

- Hippocrates

Contents

Disclaimer

Consult with your physician before you begin to participate in any workout or exercise program, including exercises in this book. I'm not a medical professional and do not claim to be. I've used all activities and advice listed within, and the described routine helped protect me from Achilles tendinitis. I have confidence in the enclosed advice and believe it will help you as it did me.

But as required in books of this type, I must state that using the guidelines included in the following pages is done at your own risk.

Introduction

Just as the strong and capable body of Achilles in Greek mythology succumbed to the single piercing of an extremity – his only weakness, his heel – you too can be felled by trauma to that small but significant part of your body. If *Achilles tendinitis* assails you, and your Achilles tendon becomes strained, inflamed, or otherwise injured, all activity dependent on this crucial link can come to a screeching halt.

The Achilles tendon is the largest and strongest tendon in the body. Regardless of its capacity to withstand the rigors of exercise – like sprinting on field and court, distance running, cardio work in the gym, or hiking – if your Achilles tendon suffers acute injury, you might be promptly sidelined from such activities. This same truth applies, sometimes to a more dire degree, if you need to stand on your feet or walk as part of earning a living.

As the connection that joins the calf muscles to the heel bone, the Achilles tendon is involved in most movements of the body when upright. This includes common motions such as running, walking, and standing. In addition, the Achilles tendon supports actions related to sports, physical work, and fitness like jumping, climbing, getting up from a crouch, and stabilizing you when you're down in that crouched position.

Achilles tendinitis is by no means rare. For example, trauma to the Achilles tendon accounts for well over 10% of running injuries. And that's just runners. Some estimates put the total incidence at well over 200,000 Achilles tendon injuries per year, in the U.S. alone. So if you suffer from Achilles tendinitis, you're far from alone. And worth a mention: if you've never been stricken by the painful setback, you can take steps in advance to prevent its arrival.

The Achilles tendinitis condition is mainly remedied with home treatment. However, surgery can be required if the Achilles tendon actually tears; if a person ignores warning signs of Achilles tendinitis for too long, and continues to perform the same high-risk activities, a complete rupture could occur. The actual causes of an Achilles tendon rupture has never been completely determined, but it's suspected that continuous injury and the resulting degeneration of the tissues play a big part. So be forewarned, and take Achilles tendinitis seriously. If ignored, it has the potential to become completely disabling. And please note, tendon tears and sutures are far beyond the scope of this book. We'll focus here on prevention of and recuperation from the much milder Achilles tendinitis.

What if you've already begun to experience the symptoms of Achilles tendinitis? You might be just starting to suspect you have the condition. Or perhaps you are already battling Achilles tendinitis and you want to accelerate the pace of improvement. If you are an athlete, and acquired Achilles tendinitis during training, you perhaps have been trying to just endure it, maintaining the usual activities and hoping it simply vanishes on its own. But so far it hasn't went away, and the pain's persisted. If that's the case, let's see if we can circumvent the nasty chain of events of partial healing and reinjury; the tips just ahead are sure to help.

How long will Achilles tendinitis stick around? Your activity level, type of work you do, weight, footwear, age, flexibility, rest periods – or lack of them – between exercise sessions, and the anatomy of your specific Achilles tendon region can all determine recuperation time. As can the length of time you've had Achilles tendinitis before you started to address it. Some folks overcome the condition in a month or less, others may heal from it over a year's time or more.

As mentioned, if you try to ignore Achilles tendinitis, and keep doing activities that brought it on to begin with, things might get worse. You could develop other maladies as well, such as knee, hip or back conditions, as you change your normal gait to favor the injury. Your best bet is to promptly take action to alleviate it and prevent its recurrence. Start the recuperation steps and preventive measures as soon as you can, and stick with them.

Maybe you've never suffered from Achilles tendinitis, but know that you're in a high-risk group: a runner, hiker, or an avid walker – especially if any of these endeavors are done on steep hills. Or perhaps you work on your feet all day, or play a sport where you sprint, stop, and start constantly. Or you're an exercise enthusiast who spends lots of time on the feet and performs forceful, quick motions. All of these groups run a higher than normal risk of acquiring Achilles tendinitis; if you're one of them, protect yourself with a stability and flexibility "force field" that will keep you standing, working, and moving with perfect functionality. The information you'll find in the upcoming pages will be just the ticket.

***

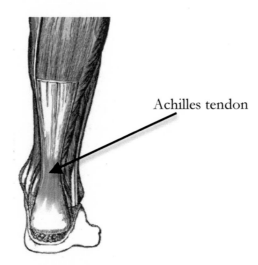

Achilles tendon

Figure 1: Location of the Achilles tendon

Characteristics

So just what is *Achilles tendinitis*? Specifically, Achilles tendinitis (also spelled Achilles *tendonitis*, either usage is correct) is severe inflammation of the Achilles tendon, the band of connective tissue (see Figure 1) that links the calf and soleus muscles of the lower leg to the heel bone. The Achilles tendon fails to function correctly when it's been subjected to numerous microscopic tears, exacerbated by limited flexibility of the person's body. With unrelenting trauma, the micro-tears that have occurred cannot heal, and the total number of these mini-injuries accumulate. Inflammation of the tendon follows and remains. The inflammation causes debilitating pain and reduced function, with a mild ache or sharp pain at the back of the lower leg and above the heel; Achilles tendinitis has set in.

Besides the tremendous workload it bears, by design the Achilles tendon is supplied with sparse blood flow, which makes it more vulnerable to injury and slower to heal.

How exactly does Achilles tendinitis get the opportunity to make you its victim? Normal wear and tear *does* contribute. The average person takes 5,000 to 12,000 steps daily. In addition to this tremendous number of footfalls, additional twists, stops, starts, and jumps a person may perform over the years can eventually tax the connective tissue of the Achilles tendon. Plus, many of the daily steps a person takes in today's world are on hard, unforgiving surfaces, and each step puts a force on the feet that is about one and a half times that person's body weight. When jogging, your feet and lower legs withstand more than three times this force. Over 10 times your body weight can be incurred while sprinting. During the course of a lifetime, the Achilles tendon tolerates immeasurable abuse as it helps and supports you as you stand, walk, and run.

Things that can tip the burden of wear and tear over the edge, resulting in the excessively repetitive or intense strain that causes Achilles tendinitis, are factors such as the following:

- Running on hard, uneven surfaces.

- Sports which involve sudden starts, stops, jumps, and surges, such as soccer, football, basketball, sprinting events, racquet sports, and more.

- Vigorous hill climbing, when either running or walking; climbing stairs fits in this category also.

- A sudden increase in the level of a running program, regarding either distance or speed.

- Wearing shoes that are worn out or of risky design.

- Lack of flexibility in the calf area.

- Embarking on intense activity with no warm-up.

- Excess body weight.

- Continuing to exert force on the injured area after warning signs appear – usually with the activities that caused the discomfort in the first place.

- Doing nothing about the swelling and inflammation of the Achilles tendon area once it begins.

– A foot with a flat arch; this can put additional duress on the Achilles tendon.

– Doing too much total exercise or work without adequate rest. In other words: overtraining and overworking.

– Outright traumatic injury to the Achilles tendon.

Any of these factors sound familiar? If any describe you, your activities, or your footwear, rest assured you're not alone. Common characteristics and behaviors can cause the condition to rear its ugly head, so you may not have done anything that horrendous or atypical to acquire Achilles tendinitis. You may have just been carrying out your exercise, work, or fitness routine, and the vulnerable link at your Achilles became affected. That's one reason it's so widespread.

How does the medical industry address Achilles tendinitis? Let's take a look, not exhaustive but rather informative, at some of the main courses of action.

Medical Procedures Related to Achilles Tendinitis

The following is a brief overview of a few methods some folks battling with Achilles tendinitis choose to undergo. This book does not advocate these treatments, it just describes them. To make an informed decision whether any of them are for you or not, consult a physician, ideally one who is familiar with sports medicine.

Corticosteroid Injections

You may be tempted to seek out a quick fix for your condition, and who wouldn't while suffering from Achilles tendinitis? That quick fix may appear to you in the form of a corticosteroid injection, which is meant to reduce swelling and pain. The injection often does just that, but its effects are usually temporary. And the temporary relief may come with grave consequences.

The majority of experts agree, corticosteroid injections can come with some nasty side effects. Some of these side effects are as follows:

– Muscle damage in the immediate area.

– Complete rupture of the tendon (as opposed to the much milder micro-tears associated with Achilles tendinitis).

– Skin pigmentation changes.

– Injury to peripheral nerves.

– Atrophy of the fat pad in your heel (padding which provides crucial protection).

Repeated injections increase these risks. What's more, the injections are not meant to fix the actual cause of your Achilles tendinitis. Use extreme caution before submitting to corticosteroid injections. If you decide to look into corticosteroid injections, you may want to get more than one doctor's opinion.

My opinion? Don't get corticosteroid injections, ever. They provide temporary relief and never actually fix soft tissue injuries; instead, they often make the injuries worse. In my own run-in with Achilles tendinitis, I personally chose to stick to conservative home care techniques instead for my bout with the condition. I preferred to address the causes of Achilles tendinitis rather than simply cover up and temporarily delay its symptoms.

Anti-Inflammatory and Pain Medication

I have strong opinions regarding the popping of pills; my feelings may rub some folks the wrong way, especially in today's somewhat medicated society. In a nutshell, I believe a person should only take pain and anti-inflammatory pills when absolutely necessary, and relying on these meds in an ongoing manner – as if they were a nutrient supplement – is pretty much denying your body's natural abilities to heal, and clutching onto a detrimental security blanket. Maybe an imaginary one at that.

Research backs up my thoughts on this issue. A recent article in the New York Times describes the findings made by exercise scientists at Appalachian State University in Boone, North Carolina. They determined that the healing of injuries to animal tissue when taking NSAIDs (non-steroidal anti-inflammatory drugs), the type of drug compound found in ibuprofen, actually *slowed* the healing of injured muscles, tendons, ligament, and bones. NSAIDs by design inhibit the production of prostaglandins, which are substances that are produced as a reaction to pain. Prostaglandins also help to create collagen, which is the building block of most tissues. So reduced creation of prostaglandins, which NSAID drugs will cause, means less collagen. This will inhibit the healing of injured tissue. Micro-tears and other trauma to muscles and tissues, as in Achilles tendinitis, fit this category.

If you and your physician decide upon medication to reduce either inflammation or pain, or both, my advice is to take as little of it as you can. As soon as the inflammation is reduced, and sharp pain turns to simple soreness, cease the medication and let your body's natural processes take over. In the case of Achilles tendinitis, let cold packs and massage (which we'll cover just ahead) take the place of pills. Of course, that's just my opinion, and it could be debated until the end of time.

Closely related: if you completely numb the pain or soreness of an injury, you may not accommodate it as much as you should with your daily motions and movement. Warning signs like pain and soreness are there for a reason. They may actually help steer you toward optimum injury recovery behavior. Don't dull your senses any more than needed.

In all types of injury recuperation, you need to address what caused the injury in the first place. Pills won't do that for you. For the most reliable, long-lasting recuperation from Achilles tendinitis, a person should stretch, strengthen, brace, and accommodate – not medicate.

Surgery

Surgery is only used for Achilles tendon trauma if a complete rupture of the tendon occurs. This book focuses on the much milder

Achilles tendinitis condition. The lesser injury, soreness, and swelling of Achilles tendinitis is sometimes the precursor to an Achilles tendon rupture, if any and all remedial and preventive steps are ignored, and activity that poses a risk to Achilles tendinitis continues.

So, as mentioned earlier, pay heed to the serious nature of Achilles tendinitis. If you do absolutely nothing else this book suggests, make sure to back off and avoid the potentially hazardous motions and situations that may have caused your Achilles tendinitis to begin with.

Extracorporeal Shockwave Therapy

Extracorporeal shockwave therapy uses ultrasound waves to encourage healing, in the hopes that the waves delivered to the affected area promote the creation of new blood vessels and result in better blood flow. It is also theorized that the brain will better "recognize" the injured area after the stimulation, and then send key nutrients to the location to further expedite healing.

It is a noninvasive procedure, so no cutting will take place. Often an ultrasound image of the injured area is taken, and the medical staff determines the greatest area of pain according to your description.

Then the treatment is delivered using a device that focuses the waves directly on the injured area. No anesthesia is necessary to complete extracorporeal shockwave therapy. Nowadays, the entire procedure can be done in the doctor's office in about 10 minutes. Extracorporeal shockwave therapy has been used now for several years to treat Achilles tendinitis, and is considered a low-risk procedure.

But please note, only a person who has experienced Achilles tendinitis for at least six months will be considered for this treatment. It can be quite costly as well. In addition, conservative, self-directed therapy as described in this book will do things extracorporeal shockwave therapy does not do: fix the factors that resulted in your condition. After all, if the underlying causes of Achilles tendinitis remain, the condition can return regardless of your undergoing this procedure or not.

***

It goes without saying, if your Achilles tendon is in trouble, so are you. There's really not a switch that gets flipped if you go to see a medical professional; you aren't likely to leave the first appointment cured. The healing process for your injury will need to be established, and then followed.

If you instead do nothing about the injury, and continue to engage in the same activities that caused your case of Achilles tendinitis, the nagging and sometimes crippling condition could remain with you for many years. Or, it could actually become chronic, in which case the malady is referred to as *Achilles tendinosis*. Sad to say, but the Achilles tendinitis condition can in some cases settle in to stay.

Don't let it. Before your athletic, fitness, or working capabilities completely collapse, take action. Don't allow it to come down to a medical procedure, as listed above, as a last resort. Luckily, some of the risk factors listed can be controlled and some behaviors changed to reduce the incidence of Achilles tendinitis and help your body heal. As a matter of fact, as mentioned, the majority of Achilles tendinitis cases are resolved through conservative home treatment, versus medical procedures or medication. Numerous preventive and recuperative maneuvers await to help you stave off Achilles tendinitis; most are rather simple and painless. You just have to learn them, and then do them. That's what we'll explore as we proceed.

Within this collection of directives, will you discover a magic formula that cures the pain of Achilles tendinitis instantly? Probably not. There's not one single, simple remedy for Achilles tendinitis; sometimes a specific motion can really provide relief, but a variety of maneuvers is usually the key. As such, we'll throw the whole kitchen sink at the condition. You'll find several tactics to reinforce the area and make the region's connections protectively strong, resilient and supple. With these motions and concepts you should enjoy a much higher degree of stability of your Achilles tendon area. Much more so than if you left its health to pure chance.

As we proceed, you will not be overwhelmed with excessive information. This book is designed for you to pick up, flip through, get some good suggestions and a dose of encouragement, and get on with the business of fixing your injury, or preventing it before it occurs. All action items are non-medical, non-invasive home treatments. They're not risky, and they should not hurt. But following these remedial steps takes perseverance. Each person is unique, as is that person's daily routine, physical condition, bodily structure, and past adventures and misadventures that have resulted in the present level of injury severity. Just a few of the action items may do the trick for you. Or you may need them all. Recuperating from Achilles tendinitis can be tricky; it's often a fine balancing act, with plenty of inaction as well as action, restraint as well as enthusiasm.

If you're burdened by an injury like Achilles tendinitis, it's hard to take the fact that your running, playing, walking, hiking, or other exercise regimen has been altered or derailed, or that you can't stay on your feet as much as your job requires. But remember that the sooner you begin, the sooner you will heal, and the more quickly you will get your capable and strong footing back.

Achilles tendinitis can be overcome. I know, as I've suffered through the condition and outmaneuvered it, using the very techniques contained in this book. If you are stricken with Achilles tendinitis, do the same. Make a surge forward and explore the full spectrum of Achilles tendinitis recuperation and prevention concepts just ahead; resolve to shun the painful condition for good. Nobody knows how long your recovery period will last, but there is definitely one best time to start it: right now.

Phase 1:
Protect and Defend

The idea of the first phase of this recovery journey is to soothe the injury and surrounding tissues, provide some relief from injury-causing agents, and create the best possible atmosphere for your Achilles to heal. After symptoms of inflammation and acute pain are reduced, it will be safer for you to proceed to the strengthening and stretching activities, which we'll cover soon.

Make a Commitment to Heal and Back Off

Let's wait on the stretching, strengthening and other physical measures for a moment. Just as important as more active rehab maneuvers is the decision to dedicate yourself to doing whatever it takes to stave off a case of Achilles tendinitis. To commit. And that commitment includes the willingness to bring certain actions to a halt if that's what it takes to get your Achilles health back.

Convincing Achilles duress to vanish is serious business; you'll have to gird yourself for the challenges ahead, and decide to dedicate a little time and effort to the endeavor. With consistency.

If you have already struggled with the condition for some time, I probably don't need to tell you to commit. If you have just started the Achilles tendinitis healing process, embrace this idea early on, and dedicate yourself to your recovery.

You'll need every advantage you can get. After all, you cannot perform your healing process in a vacuum. You still need to walk. You may need to stand on your feet for long periods of time. You still get back on your feet after a night spent in bed, and still get in and out of a tub or shower. And each of these and numerous other actions can cause a slight reinjury to your Achilles; as the reinjuries accumulate, your malady can be prevented from healing in short order. So, you must consistently do many positive things while keeping the negative factors to an absolute minimum. The more the odds can be tipped in your favor, the better.

Most people cannot stay off their feet indefinitely, and this probably includes you. And even if you could, the weakened state of your feet and legs as a result of this inactivity would end up making matters worse. You must keep moving and stay strong, yet stave off backward progress. Therein lies the complex puzzle that is recuperation from Achilles tendinitis. The balance required to reduce the condition and heal from it makes for a delicate scenario.

You've acquired a condition that has no fix-it pill, no miracle cure, no definite recovery time line, and no single cause that can be blamed for its existence. And Achilles tendinitis has a nasty habit of recurring once normal activities are resumed. It's going to take a serious commitment from you to bring your Achilles tendon back to a normal, uninjured condition. And then keep it there.

If you don't take Achilles tendinitis seriously at first, and push through the warning signs or try to ignore them, you could add weeks or months to your recovery phase. Don't make this mistake. Now is not the time to become complacent regarding your course of action for recovery.

Study the action items included in this book, and follow them with consistency. As mentioned already, you may need just a few of the actions to make a full recovery, or you may need every single one. Each person is unique, so your recovery plan may be somewhat individualized. You might recover from your injury quickly, maybe in just a few weeks. Or it may take you months, or maybe a year or more. Thousands of victims of Achilles tendinitis have proven that lengthy recoveries are fairly common; others have proven the condition can go away almost overnight. I'm willing to bet that a large percentage of the slow-to-heal victims delayed taking action to rectify their injuries. Or just as risky, they jumped back into full, rigorous activity too soon.

If you're bummed, try to fend off the doom and gloom. Recovery happens. Admit to yourself the serious nature of the situation that has befallen you, and immerse yourself in the process needed for recovery. Take action right away, be confident, be patient, be consistent, and your injury will heal much faster.

For the speediest recovery from Achilles tendinitis, you must stop doing the activity that you suspect caused it in the first place, or at least reduce that activity as much as possible. If only ceasing activity was that easy. If you love to hike or take long walks, turning your back on these activities can be difficult to endure. If you are a dedicated runner or exercise enthusiast, shelving a program can be grueling. You may feel pent up, cooped up, restless, and unfulfilled. To hang up your exercise ritual, even for a short time, may be unthinkable.

If you work on your feet, you face an even more complex scenario. In some ways, your feet are your fortune, and when adjusting a schedule and job duties with a boss and team members you may or may not experience a smooth transition.

But you must reduce the wear and tear on your Achilles tendon, and that may mean making some tough choices and significant changes to a routine. At least temporarily. If you do not, you'll most likely hinder progress toward your recovery. Grind away as in the past, continue stubbornly ahead even when it hurts, and wear the same hazardous footwear that you've been wearing, and the Achilles tendinitis condition may in fact never heal.

Blessedly, Achilles tendinitis sometimes improves greatly just from extended rest. But that usually takes "intervention" from you to help it along. By doing less, often way less. In other words, veer away from the causative activities as best possible, and rest up. Easier said than done in many cases, but crucial for healing. Make an unwavering commitment to help yourself heal, and you'll get that stable footing back under you as soon as possible.

Wear Protective Shoes

You will need to plant your feet in a supportive, durable, resilient pair of shoes as soon as possible to minimize further damage or irritation to your Achilles. Once you've got the shoe piece of the puzzle figured out, you'll have made great strides in activating the healing process. Good shoes can protect your feet and lower legs like a dream, and bad ones can sabotage them like a nightmare. In fact, dangerous shoes may have landed you on the Achilles tendinitis "injured reserve" list in the first place.

Although a sales rep at a reputable shoe store can help you work out the details, here are a few things to look for as you seek new footwear:

- **Flexibility.** Make sure the shoe bends in the front half, where the ball of the foot will be when the shoe is worn. It should not bend in the middle or way back closer to the heel. Your shoe should not bend in any area where your foot does not normally bend. If it does, that shoe's support will be marginal. Conversely, if the shoe barely bends at all, rule it out as an overly-stiff shoe that will be detrimental to your feet and Achilles tendon.

- **Stiff Heel Counter.** The back of the shoe where it engulfs your heel should fit firm and snug. Make sure your heel doesn't slide up and down.

- **Proper Fit for Your Feet...Right Now.** Have your feet measured before purchasing your next pair of shoes. Like most parts of our bodies, the feet change with age and the rigors of time. The current shoe size you need may be different than what you wore in the past. The width of your feet should be measured in addition to their length.

- **Arch Support.** Sufficient backbone where the shoe supports your arch is critical. Ensure that the shoe is not flimsy in this area and does not flatten out as you walk.

- **Low Heel.** This one is obvious. No more high heels or dashing boots that jack the back of your foot way up. Lose the pointy toes also.

- **A Little Room to Move.** You'll want a small amount of space in your shoes, both in terms of length and width, so your feet will be comfortable and blood can flow easily. Make sure your new shoes are not too roomy but not too tight either. This is especially important as the day progresses, since your feet will swell slightly as time goes on. As a matter of fact, for this very reason the best time to try on a pair of shoes is later in the day.

- **A Design Matching High-Arched or Low-Arched Feet.** If you have a low arch, your foot type will benefit from a more rigid shoe with "motion control" design. If you have a high arch, your foot type is somewhat stiff and requires more cushioning – but not too much! Those shoes with extreme cushioning, like the type with inflated air pockets lifting the shoe way up, are actually a risk factor for Achilles problems. Due to this shoe construction, as the heel makes contact, it continues to sink lower than it should, stretching the already-stressed tendon further. Avoid this design.

- **A Good Fit and Feel Immediately.** A pair of shoes that aligns correctly with your feet should feel comfortable upon trying them on. Don't assume that the shoes will break in and accommodate your feet with time. They probably won't.

Make sure to replace your worn out shoes. Yes, even your favorite ones. Favorite old shoes, even those with no support left in them, can be set aside for a while and then somehow find their way back onto injured, recuperating legs. Acquiring new, solid-performing shoes is half of the footwear equation. Banish the old faithful but beat up shoes; they can put your Achilles tendon back in danger. Throw them away if they appear to be mostly degraded. If they seem to be in usable condition but not intact enough for serious exercise, you can give them away to charity and still feel good about parting ways with them. And they may in fact work for someone else just fine. It could be that those shoes are just not right for your feet and circumstances.

For runners, some experts recommend replacing shoes every 500 miles. Other experts say replace them every 300 or 400 miles. For walkers, add about 100 miles to these figures at most. The owner of an old and loyal pair can generally tell if support from those shoes is expiring. If you have a pair of shoes that have served you well, but fit the description of "waning support," make your peace, bid them farewell, and get yourself some new ones. Give your Achilles and all related muscles, tissues, and joints a new start.

Experiment with Heel Cups

You may want to supplement your new robust, highly protective shoes with a pair of heel cups. A heel cup can be used inside your shoes to control excessive pronation (this is when the foot comes down on its inner margin or instep), and can be a positive addition to a program of Achilles tendonitis recuperation.

A heel cup is simply an insert that is placed in the back of your shoe, to add cushioning and lift your heel a bit. The slight lift (I'm not advocating adding an entire inch to your height here) a heel cup provides may relieve some of the tension your Achilles tendon undergoes, and spare it from excessive stretching. This relief will set up a better environment for recuperation.

In addition, the cup will supply some mild cushioning. The human foot is equipped with a padding of fat covering the heel. This padding protects your foot against impact and wear. With time, rigor, and age, however, the padding begins to spread out, and some of its shock-absorbing effectiveness is lost. A heel cup will help compensate for this diminished natural protection. It may also supply some cushioning which a given pair of shoes does not have. This additional relief to your heel will reduce wear and tear to your Achilles tendon in turn.

Heel cups can be purchased over the counter, and most every pharmacy and department store seems to carry at least one brand. These orthotic inserts are inexpensive, easily acquired and surprisingly helpful for some people. These simple devices can relieve discomfort, promote healing, and in the future ward off a recurrence of Achilles tendinitis.

Heel cups may help a little or help a lot. Very little risk is involved in experimenting with them. Note: the tightness of your shoes may need to be adjusted after adding a heel cup. You may want to loosen the laces a bit to accommodate the new protective layer in your shoes. Other than that, place the insert in your shoes, and you're ready to go.

Give a pair of heel cups a try and see what you think. They just might lend some immediate relief, reinforce the natural protection your body provides, and help prevent ongoing Achilles pain.

Adjust Your Training and Exercise Routine

It will be a complete judgment call as to the level of activity you maintain if you become stricken with Achilles tendinitis. Only one thing is certain: if you believe you were waylaid by overexertion, as runners and hikers with Achilles tendinitis generally are, then you need to cut back on your activity.

How much to reduce your normal routine? Nobody can tell you for sure, but if your Achilles area is inflamed and sore to the touch, it's probably not a bad idea to do next to nothing for a while. Not a popular statement in endurance athlete circles, but…it may be necessary.

I've come across the advice numerous times that the individual suffering Achilles tendinitis should cut activity just a bit, like by a mere 10% or so. To that I say dream on. Not trying to be snarky here, but a 10% reduction is pretty light duty. If that's all you need to cut back to become healthy again, I'd think you didn't have a really serious situation in the first place. If, on the other hand, you are wincing when walking, cannot run at all or climb a hill without pain, and your Achilles area is tender to the touch, it's in your interest to reduce rigorous activity, either mostly or completely. Think for the long-term, and don't make a case of tendinitis into a permanent condition.

In terms of **prevention**, here are some important rules to follow:

Avoid sudden increases in training:

This is a case where the 10% rule is preached again, but I think it applies here more readily. Regardless of the type of training or activity you do, it's advised by many coaches and fitness trainers to never increase your training by increments greater than 10%. This applies to duration, distance, and intensity. A very good rule to follow, in my opinion.

And I'll go as far as to say consider increasing your training quantity in even smaller amounts. Athletes and exercisers don't always have to go for "longer, better, faster." Consistency and staying power are often much more important than continually stepping it up. Go with training and activity increases of less than 10%, and you'll be sure to not overwhelm your adaptation to exercise amounts.

If you often walk or run a three-mile route, just add a 200-yard distance or a city block now and then, if anything. If you're used to working out on a treadmill for 45:00, don't think you have to add 4:30 (10%) to your session if you decide to step it up. Just add a minute or two at a time. Be sensible and work up at a modest pace. Your odds of suffering Achilles tendinitis will then be lessened.

Avoid excessive hill running:

Or, related to the above concept, suddenly adding hills and inclines to your regimen. Very few things pose the risk of acquiring Achilles tendinitis as walking, hiking, and especially running up steep hills. Aggressive inclines and flights of stairs apply here too. Keep this in mind as you look to prevent the injury from cropping up.

I love running up hills and steep inclines. It almost makes for the perfect endurance and fitness workout: it increases intensity without the horrendous pounding of a sprint on flat ground, and it builds strength, as if your lower body was being worked with weights as you run. Those facts make the Achilles tendinitis risk of navigating hills and inclines a sad paradox.

The answer: storm hills and flights of stairs in moderation, work up to a given duration over time, and ideally perform a thorough warm-up before you tackle these workouts and routes. In addition, bolster your defenses with the stretching and strengthening motions we'll cover soon.

Maintain Low Impact Form

In addition to becoming stronger and more flexible, you'll want to minimize one of the primary enemies of your feet and Achilles tendons: impact. Here are some ways to do that.

Shorten your stride, whether walking, running, or just moving about. Changing the length with which you step can seem awkward at first, but a short time after consciously adjusting your stride you'll most likely stick to it for good. A short stride feels more efficient and actually helps you move forward faster. It will feel better on your feet and heels. And it will decrease your chance of an additional cumulative stress injury.

A heavy heel strike results from a long, reaching stride. More impact on your feet and lower leg is the outcome. A lengthy stride can result in more soreness in your knees, hamstrings, quadriceps, and shins. It is inefficient and actually wastes energy. And the added impact will be brutal on your lower legs. This can really add up if you run, as running produces impact several times your body weight. Although the stress will be realized more intensely if you run, the force upon your heels can be about 1.5 times your body weight even when walking. As opposed to a long, lumbering stride, a shorter stride benefits you when walking also, as it helps minimize the force of impact.

Besides using a shorter stride, practice an ideal foot strike. When either walking or running, you may find it tempting to land on the balls of your feet, or even on your tiptoes. It would stand to reason, since sharp pain emanates from your heels, to keep contact with the ground as far from your heels as possible. However, you should avoid this urge. When you land on the balls of your feet or your tiptoes, you actually stress the Achilles tendon *more*, not less. The stress realized during any long walks or distance running while landing on your tiptoes will be felt immediately. And it won't feel pleasant.

Similarly, you should avoid walking or running on the outside edges of your feet. This foot placement will not let the foot roll forward as it was meant to, and like landing on your tiptoes, will probably compound your injury.

You should still land on your heel with each step – ideally toward the *front* of the heel, right around the middle of the foot. Landing on the middle of the foot goes along with a shorter, controlled stride, and results in better shock absorption. You avoid the excessive force from a strike at the very back of the heel, which is all but impossible to avoid if your stride is more like a long, exaggerated lunge.

Even if you feel a little soreness, let the foot roll forward as it does during non-injured walking and running. Landing with the middle of the foot will assist with an ideal rolling forward motion. And remember, good shoes should protect the injured area of your heels to a large extent. So again, make sure you wear good shoes.

And finally, glide with your feet, don't thump. Let your feet skim just above the ground with each step. Don't raise way up and pound the foot down with each step. If you're one of the countless people who walk and run like this (I myself was one), now is the time to adjust the forceful landing you inflict upon your feet.

I know of what I speak here, because I was one of the greatest offenders. For years, I would bound along when running, reaching as far as I could with each leg. My lead foot would fly way above the ground, and then crash down upon landing. My legs and feet would take a terrible pounding, but I persisted with this self-defeating stride. I actually trained for and ran numerous 8K and 10K races this way. In fact, during downhill sections of some courses, I would leap up and out as much as possible with each step, letting myself become airborne for a moment before crushing impact met each footfall. I figured, why not just let gravity take me? And I wondered why my shins were on fire and my hamstring muscles almost nonfunctional with soreness for days afterward. Not to mention, it seemed like the runners whom I had burst past on the downhill portion, the ones with more relaxed, controlled strides, always seemed to pass me up a short time later. It took a painful bout of Achilles tendinitis to make me step back and examine what I was doing wrong.

Having trouble picturing what I mean here? If you've ever watched a major league baseball game, and saw the defenders make a key third out, or better yet a double play, you may have seen the players then proudly bound off the field. Way up, way down, loping along with vitality, thundering down with each step of their heroic all-star jog. It looks impressive, and it's actually kind of fun to run that way.

But if your Achilles tendons are in the process of healing, restrain yourself. Looking good and feeling good can be two different things. Be good to your legs, be good to your knees, and be good to your feet. Keep your stride short. Contact with your midfoot. Keep your feet low to the ground, whisking them along and planting them quickly but gently. You'll walk and run with more efficiency, move just as fast if not faster than before, and expose your body to far less damaging impact.

Avoid Dangerous Surfaces

In short, be careful where you walk and run. Some hazards are obvious. Others can disguise themselves better, and may even look inviting.

Icy areas represent probably the most evident example of a dangerous surface. With your feet slipping, sliding, gliding, and floating unpredictably in any direction, icy surfaces can inflict extra damage to your already tender Achilles tendon. And on those flat icy areas with ice and snow chunks frozen in place, walking can be horrific. Don't attempt to navigate ice-covered areas unless you absolutely have to.

Moving across any type of surface that is uneven will be questionable to the safety of your lower legs. Luckily, walking in such an area will feel uncomfortable, and you'd probably sense that it's not good for your Achilles area. And you'd be right. The foot in the lower position is subject to undue stress, as it carries an excessive proportion of the load in this situation. Choose relatively even surfaces if you can.

But what about a nice sandy beach, or the local park's big, green expanse of grass? Proceed with caution. Both of these surfaces can actually stress the Achilles tendon to a great degree. Walking or running in soft, sandy areas can be deceptively rough on your feet. Trudging in the sand will often result in the heel plunging below the level of the forefoot at the moment your weight comes to bear over your entire foot. While the heel is in this negative position, it experiences far more pressure than when walking on level ground: the additional force can actually be three or four times greater. A sandy surface may look alluring, but watch out.

Grassy areas pose a mixed scenario: grass has some positive aspects and some negative ones too. The cushion grass provides is undeniable, and it's mostly a good thing. Not much brutal impact will be realized on grass. On the other hand, lawns and fields of grass are inevitably uneven. Bumps, dips, pieces of litter, roots, and rocks can lie hidden anywhere in grass. As can actual holes made by rodents. So despite the padding grass provides, it is not an optimum surface on which to walk or run when recovering from Achilles tendinitis.

And of course, we all know the reality of unyielding concrete, as that's what most sidewalks consist of. Concrete is unforgiving, absorbing almost no shock from your footfalls. Much better choices for walking are dirt, gravel or wood chip paths, providing they are even and in good condition. Asphalt is actually not a bad surface either, specifically in warm weather. It becomes somewhat shock-absorbing as the sun heats it and makes it soft. In extreme cold, however, it becomes as unforgiving as concrete.

Beware of hills as well. Like grassy surfaces, traveling on hills contains desirable and not so desirable aspects. The vigorous climbs and descents steep hills provide can build strength, endurance, and muscle tone to a great degree, especially in the very leg muscles you need to solidify for future injury protection. Unfortunately, when traveling uphill, the ankle is forced into what is called *dorsiflexion.* Dorsiflexion means the foot bends back so your toes are closer to your shin. While in this position, the Achilles tendon is getting stretched, and in some cases strained, as it bears the weight of the rest of your body being heaved up the hill. On the downhill trip, the ankle goes into the opposite position, *plantar flexion.* The plantar flexion position results in a similar foot strike as when walking on the balls of your feet (or high heels), which is detrimental to the feet at any time, but especially when recovering from Achilles tendinitis. Add to the fact that your body weight is pounding down with extra momentum thanks to gravity on your downhill descent, and the result is a significant load for your injured lower legs to bear. Walking and especially running on hills can be rough on an Achilles tendinitis sufferer.

Is there any way to limit the strain from traveling up and down hills? I found one strategy helps above all else: keep your stride short. Don't reach way up when going uphill. And don't step big and allow your weight to crash down on your leading foot on the downhill descent. Landing on your midfoot will help also, as it keeps your foot more level, and diminishes the extreme positions of dorsiflexion and plantar flexion. If you keep your stride short, striking on the midfoot is much easier to accomplish.

Are you expected to maneuver on completely flat and perfectly forgiving surfaces at all times? Of course not. That would be difficult if not impossible to achieve as you move through your day or go for walks in various areas. Hard or slippery surfaces, small hills, and short but steep inclines occur in most areas, and you can travel on them to a limited extent without a problem. The key to remember is the concept of *cumulative stress*. Achilles tendinitis results because of stress, strain, wear and tear occurring over and over from certain damaging factors. Try to avoid risky areas and steep hills if you can, and certainly don't plan to exercise on them.

Ice the Injured Area

The Achilles tendinitis condition is an injury, and like most injuries, swelling occurs in the immediate area. This inflammation will not only increase discomfort, it will limit normal motion and impede the healing process. The most immediate and effective method to reduce the inflammation is to apply ice to the injury. Ice will enhance your healing and deaden some of the pain. It will help remove detrimental fluids and allow nutrients to enrich the injured site. This will encourage the repair process and help your heels heal sooner.

Various methods are available to deliver ice applications to the injury, such as commercial ice packs, a plastic bottle filled with water and allowed to freeze, or ice cubes wrapped in a towel. Another good and very convenient method is simply a bag of frozen vegetables. Frozen corn kernels and peas are both ideal, as their rounded shape makes for a comfortable texture when you do the icing. The individual pieces in the bag move freely and will mold to the shape of your lower leg. And the bags can be used over and over.

The procedure can be as easy as placing the frozen veggies on the floor, then resting your Achilles area on them as you sit in a comfortable chair. Unless it causes pain, you can work a gentle ice massage into the treatment by moving your lower leg against the ice pack, slowly and gently. Another common technique is to wrap an ice pack in a towel, then rest your legs on that cold source.

Do not apply ice or frozen items directly against your skin. This can cause ice burns and damage to your skin. Place a moist towel between your skin and the cold pack to avoid any such danger.

Do not overdo it with icing. Ice treatment of the tender area for 10 minutes at a given time is usually plenty. You can actually damage the tissue if you ice it excessively. Do the icing twice a day in the early stage of Achilles tendinitis, or if a reinjury of your Achilles area ever crops up. Once you're well on your way to healing, once a day should be enough.

Icing will be especially valuable if you have just been on your feet for a long time, or right after walking or running. Do it immediately following these activities for best results.

Speaking of walking, running, and reinjury: if you do at some point jump back into activity with a little too much vigor and suffer a reinjury, make sure to apply ice to the area as soon as you can. The benefit of icing an acute injury diminishes after 48 hours or so. Catch the recurrence in time with ice treatment, and the damage will be greatly minimized.

Keep icing in mind for a convenient, low cost, and effective form of therapy. Sit back, relax, and let your aching Achilles region chill a bit.

Phase 2:
Stretch and Strengthen

- A Word About Stretching -

For starters, do not stretch any part of the Achilles region if acute pain exists, or if sharp pain results from stretching motions. If you are in the acute stages of Achilles tendinitis, where the area is painful to the touch, it may be too early to implement stretching in your action plan. Wait until rest and protection let the area start to recuperate, then try some of the stretches listed with caution in mind. And, just as importantly, if you think you're up for stretching, but a given motion causes sharp pain, cease it immediately. You may not be ready yet.

No absolute verdict has ever been reached on the very best method with which to stretch portions of the human body. If you had the will and unlimited time, and researched the topic until locating 100 articles or books on stretching, I think you would find some glaring discrepancies. It's easy to find 25 or 50 or 60 different takes on the number of repetitions, length of time to hold a stretch, stretching a cold muscle vs. a warmed-up muscle, and how far to stretch an inflexible muscle. Overwhelming agreement amongst the experts on stretching does not seem to exist. And I don't have the final answer on stretching, but I know a couple of things:

Stretching can help you recover from Achilles tendinitis, and
Stretching can INJURE you further.

Over the years of running races and training, I got into the bad habit of never stretching. My best guess is that this lack of stretching helped me acquire Achilles tendinitis in the first place. But once I started stretching on a regular basis, the healing process accelerated - greatly. The healing seemed to take place several times faster. And on walks and hikes where the soreness would recur, taking the time to stretch again would usually reduce the pain or make it go away completely. Stretching is a good thing, and most experts on the subject agree that it is not only helpful, but imperative, to stretch to resolve a case of Achilles tendinitis.

So let me reiterate: I'm all for stretching. A stretching routine helped me heal from Achilles tendinitis and earlier an even worse case of plantar fasciitis, and it keeps my feet and heels safe to this day. Stretching is an integral part of this book and can serve as an invaluable healing mechanism for anyone who suffers from or wants to prevent Achilles tendinitis.

But if you stretch a muscle with too much force and in too much of a hurry, the muscle can tear. And your injury problem will then become compounded. So keep three words in mind for a successful stretching venture:

Consistent. Patient. Gentle.

When overcoming a case of Achilles tendinitis, only perform the stretches after warming up. A slow walk that gradually increases to medium speed generally works.

Stretch regularly, at least once a day, as you help yourself heal from Achilles tendinitis. A couple of times a week will not be enough. And try not to hurry. You must hold a stretch for it to work, and you might find yourself becoming a bit bored. Practice patience. And above all, be gentle when stretching. If it hurts, back off. If a stretch goes no further without discomfort, don't force the stretch past that point. Ever. Be gentle and you won't injure yourself while stretching.

How long should you hold a stretch? Over the years I've heard figures from two seconds all the way up to sixty seconds, and a wide variety within that range. Basically, they've all worked for me. As long as I did the stretches in the first place, and didn't get too rough while doing them. I've listed the very general estimate in this book of holding a stretch 10-20 seconds, then repeating that stretch three or four times. Why? It's worked for the masses over time, and is a good general rule of thumb. If you find holding a stretch shorter or longer than 10-20 seconds works better, then do it that way. Experiment and find the best duration of stretching for you personally.

Just remember to be consistent, patient, and gentle, and your stretching endeavor will be effective.

Stretch Your Calf Muscles

Flexibility in your calf muscles is crucial to reducing the injured condition of your heel; its importance cannot be overstated. The calf muscle works incredibly hard any time you walk or run; in the human body, only the heart muscle does more work than the calf. So lack of flexibility in the calf will cause unwelcome wear on your body day after day. Limberness in this area is vital to recovery from Achilles tendinitis.

The repetitive impact from motions like running and walking eventually causes your related muscles and tendons to become short and tight. This is already hard on the Achilles tendon, and a tight calf area stresses it even more.

Tight calf muscles pull on the Achilles tendon, exerting quite a strain on it. While under this increased tension, the introduction of any of the other factors which contribute to Achilles tendinitis (bad shoes, excessive exercise, excessive weight, hazardous surfaces, etc.) exacerbates the damage. Already embattled with the duress, the Achilles tendon undergoes extra strain and impact from tightness in the calf. Tight calf muscles interfere with normal foot and leg mechanics, and your Achilles tendon suffers as a consequence. Repeated pounding on short, tight muscles can cause micro-tears in the tendon.

The combination of inflexible calves with other risk factors can often lead to a full-blown case of Achilles tendinitis. In contrast, the introduction of flexibility in the calves removes a big liability for getting the condition in the first place. If you already suffer from it, Achilles tendinitis is less likely to stick around once your calf area becomes flexible. So we have to stretch that area, and make it supple and forgiving; make your calves more limber to reduce the strain on your Achilles tendon.

Remember: think gentle. You're stretching the very region that is injured, so take care to not worsen the condition by stretching too vigorously. That said, you might find yourself amazed at the reduction in tenderness and the return of durability your Achilles region will experience once flexibility in the calf area gets established. Dedicate yourself to this simple stretching routine and realize big dividends.

First and Foremost: Avoid the World's Worst Calf Stretch

If you value the living tissues in your body, never, ever perform the stretch I'll describe shortly. But first let me say that with regard to stretching, as with most things, there is advice. Then there is questionable advice. And then there is *insane* advice. Case in point:

Floating about the Achilles tendinitis and plantar fasciitis rehab community is one very risky, aggressive, and hazardous stretching technique. This is probably the most common stretch a person with either condition will be recommended...and ironically, the stretch is horribly dangerous. It goes as follows:

Stand on a step, curb, or ledge of some kind, putting your weight on the ball of the foot to be stretched (Figure 2).

Then, the advisors of this stretch say, lower that heel way down, letting all of your bodyweight pile on to stretch out your calf area.

This is to be done, according to those advisors, on one already tender, injured foot and/or Achilles tendon...with your full body weight. Bad idea. (I couldn't bring myself to fully demonstrate this tactic in Figure 2; I kept a little weight on my front foot to avoid a painful re-tearing. In most instances where this stretch is recommended, however, the "expert" instructs the person to stand fully on the injured foot. Ouch!)

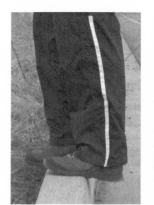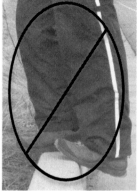

Figure 2: World's worst calf stretch starting position (left picture) and ending position (right picture)

My oh my. I can almost feel the vulnerable tissue give way a little more, exacerbating the injury further. A forceful, brutal, impatient stretch like this is the *last* thing you want to do when you are recovering from Achilles tendinitis. A soft tissue recovery routine should be more like walking on eggshells, not squashing grapes into wine, if you catch my drift. **Do NOT** perform the stretch as detailed above.

Let's try a similar and much safer version of this stretch. As demonstrated in Figure 3, standing next to the step or curb, place the ball of your foot to be stretched against the structure. (You could place the heel of your foot on the floor and the ball of it against a wall for that matter.) Keep most of your weight on your supporting leg, not the leg to be stretched. This allows you to control the intensity of the stretch, and carry it out as all stretches should be carried out: *gently*.

Proceed to lean ever so slowly into the stretch. Hold it at the point the stretch first starts; do not stretch beyond that point. Hold it 10-20 seconds. Repeat this process once or twice. Do this twice a day. You'll realize an effective stretch which you can control, which can be done almost anywhere, and which causes you no further harm.

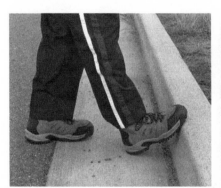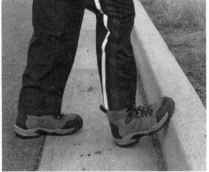

Figure 3: Answer to the "world's worst calf stretch" starting position (left picture) and ending position (right picture)

So there's a bad stretch adjusted to become a good one. Let's look at some more.

Seated Calf Stretch

While sitting on a comfortable surface, extend both legs in front of you. Reach forward carefully and grab your toes and the balls of your feet. (You can bend your knees as necessary; the stretch still works with bent knees.) Ever so mildly, pull the top of your foot back toward you, to the point that you feel a stretch begin. You should feel the effect in your calf and in the Achilles tendon at the back of the heel. Pull no further; hold that position and let the stretch take place.

If you presently have some difficulty reaching your feet in this position, as many people do, first wrap a towel around the bottom of your feet, then extend your legs in front of you (see Figure 4). With this extra reach in place, proceed with the calf stretch in the same way as described above. Position the towel around the balls of your feet, and initiate the stretch with a light touch. Once you feel the stretch take effect, stretch no further and hold it at that point.

Maintain the stretch for 10-20 seconds, and repeat the process three or four times.

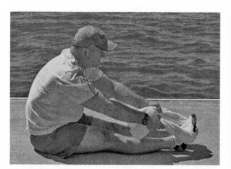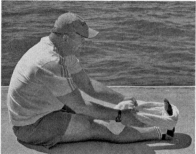

Figure 4: Seated calf stretch using a towel; starting position (left picture) and stretched position (right picture)

Wall Calf Stretch

This stretch shines due to both its effectiveness and its versatility. You won't need to don special exercise clothes or lie down on the floor. It can be done at almost any time regardless of what you're wearing, and just about anywhere that a wall exists. Furthermore, items like a chest of drawers, a chair, or even a large tree can be used in place of a wall. The ready availability of the wall stretch makes it ideal to do while out on a walk, at work, or before and after any exercise session.

Place your hands on the wall, and the leg to be stretched set back behind you, foot flat on the floor (see Figure 5). The front leg will be slightly bent at the knee. T o execute the stretch, let your forward leg flex a bit more at the knee, and maneuver your hips slightly forward. Gently move into the stretch. Once you feel the stretch in the calf area and the Achilles tendon (at the back of the heel) go no further and hold the stretch. Hold for 10-20 seconds. Repeat the sequence three or four times.

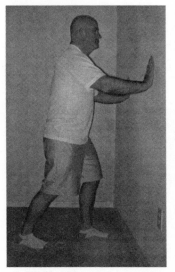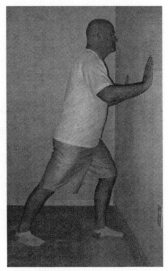

Figure 5: Wall calf stretch starting position (left picture) and stretched position (right picture)

Wall Soleus Stretch

The idea here, in part, is to stretch the soleus muscle, the strong layer of muscle which lies underneath your calf muscles. Flexibility here will ease tension on the Achilles, just as calf flexibility does.

Stand facing a wall with feet about shoulder width apart. Place both hands on the wall at about chest level and brace yourself. Then bend both knees just a little bit, put your right foot forward, and keep both feet flat on the floor (see Figure 6). Lean toward the wall. Be gentle with this motion. Wait until you feel a stretch in your lower calf area, then hold it there a few seconds. While you're doing this, keep the heel of your left foot on the floor. This will stretch the calf muscle of the left leg at the same time the soleus muscle of the right is stretched.

Reverse feet, and perform the stretch that way. Repeat in each direction two or three times for a good stretch of your lower leg muscles.

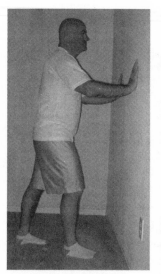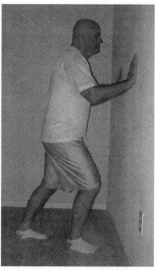

Figure 6: Soleus stretch starting position (left picture) and stretched position (right picture)

Stretch Your Arches Plus

In addition to stretching out your calf area to reduce strain on the Achilles tendon, you can stretch the arch itself. This will make the Achilles tendon slightly more flexible, reducing the pulling and strain experienced where it attaches at the heel. The result will be reduced tenderness and less swelling in the heel and arch. (This is also a great stretch for your plantar fascia.)

The procedure for the arch stretch is as follows: while sitting, set your lower leg on your opposite knee. Grab your toes and the ball of your foot, and gently bend the foot back (see Figure 7). If you are in the early throes of the Achilles tendinitis ordeal, don't expect to bend your foot back very far before you feel some soreness. Stop the stretch if you feel pain at any point. Ease up, and stretch your arch to a lesser degree. If you attempt to stretch the arch further than it's ready to be stretched, you could injure yourself further. Developing flexibility anywhere in the body is a gradual process, and nowhere is this truer than in the arch. Hold the stretch for about 10-20 seconds, and repeat the process three or four times.

I recommend doing this stretch a little later in the morning instead of first thing upon awakening. All parts of your body will be stiffened from sleep, especially your arch. You may want to move around for a while and then do the arch stretch. Your foot, ankle, and heel area will then be warmed up from stepping and walking, and may be more safely stretched. If you do decide to stretch your arches early in the morning, before walking, do so with extra care. Slow motion and ultra-gentle would be the idea in that case.

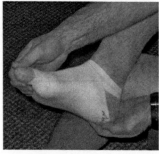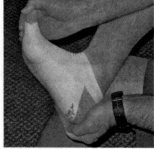

Figure 7: Arch Plus stretch starting position (left picture) and stretched position (right picture)

Stretch Your Hamstrings

Tight hamstrings can be tough to live with. Not only do inflexible hamstrings put these long, strong muscles in the back of your thighs themselves at risk, but they also cause undue tension on other body parts. The most publicized by-product of stiff hamstrings is the extra wear and tear they cause on the lower back. Similarly, tight hamstrings place extra stress on the Achilles tendon.

It's a somewhat complex series of events. Lack of hamstring flexibility can cause less-than-ideal leg motions. One example is over-flexion of the knee. When the knee over-flexes, the effect travels down the leg, and excess flexion of the ankle increases as well. This then exerts extra pull on the heel bone and Achilles tendon; this can contribute to Achilles tendinitis occurring and staying.

In addition, flexible and strong hamstring muscles assist in dissipating the force that travels throughout the leg when walking or running. When they're overly tight, the hamstrings can't do their part in this impact reduction.

Simply put, like tight calf muscles and Achilles tendons, inflexible hamstrings are quite taxing on the Achilles tendon. And allowing them to stay inflexible means the progress in your recovery will be hindered.

A number of good hamstring stretches are out there, and here's one that is effective, safe, and somewhat relaxing.

While on your back, raise one leg, keeping it bent at the knee just a bit, hold the leg behind the knee, and slowly, gently extend your leg (see Figure 8). This will stretch the hamstring area. Expect the hamstring to be a little tight if you have not stretched it regularly.

A slight variation to this procedure is to wrap a towel around the center of your foot, versus holding your leg with your hands. Pull carefully on the towel as you extend your leg, stopping and holding the position once you feel a stretch begin.

Hold the stretch for about 10-20 seconds, and repeat the process three or four times.

Of all the endeavors listed in this book, developing hamstring flexibility is one of the most beneficial to your entire body. It assists in ease of movement in just about every motion your body can perform, in both your exercise routine and your daily tasks. And it feels good, almost a relief, when tight hamstrings get good and loosened up.

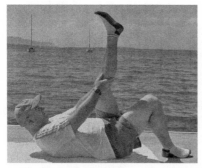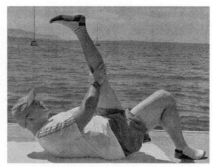

Figure 8: Supine hamstring stretch starting position (left picture) and stretched position (right picture)

Strengthen Your Calf and Achilles Area

To help stabilize the motion of your ankles and feet, work on building strength in your calf muscles and the interrelated Achilles region. Strong muscles in your calf area assist in controlling the action of the foot's strike, roll, and push-off with each step. The stronger your calves are, the more your Achilles and feet will be stabilized during this process.

Strengthening your calf muscles will deliver the extra benefit of greater endurance: you'll be able to work, exercise and stand in place longer without tiring your lower legs. Your Achilles in turn will receive better support and protection. This will make things like maintaining weight (through exercise), getting through a workday on your feet, and having fun outdoors more attainable.

Your calves get worked during just about any movement you make on your feet or with your legs. Walking, biking, running, playing tennis, and climbing stairs are just a few examples of activities which involve your calf muscles, as well as many other muscles simultaneously. To focus on the calves, you can use just a few simple yet effective exercises. Aim to do them every other day or so; a day or two of rest in between exercise sessions will allow for muscle recovery. The motions are as follows:

Seated Calf Raise

This exercise can be performed either with or without additional resistance. Using no additional resistance will work on the endurance of the calf muscle, while adding some weights (resistance) will increase the strength. While seated with your feet resting directly in front of you, place your hands at your sides or on your knees (see Figure 9). Now simply raise your heels up off the ground. Keep doing the motion until exhaustion sets in, and then stop.

If you prefer to work on the strength of the calf muscle, rest a towel or padding of some kind across your knees. On top of the towel or padding place a weight, a barbell plate for instance, and then again simply raise your heels up off the ground. Keep doing the motion until exhaustion sets in, and then stop.

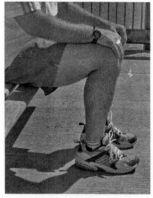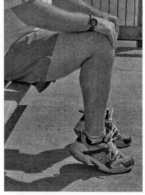

Figure 9: Seated calf raise starting position (left picture) and flexed position (right picture)

In place of a barbell plate, you could use a different form of resistance, such as a pair of phone books. Or, you could actually push down on your knees with the palms of your hands, supplying the resistance with your upper body strength. Your imagination is the only limit here.

If you've not been exercising regularly in recent times, just complete one set with this exercise as well. Add another set or two later if and when you feel ready.

Standing Calf Raise

There's not a lot to describe here; while standing, raise yourself up so your heels leave the ground, and you balance on the balls of your feet (see Figure 10). Lower your heels back down, and you have just completed one repetition. Continue with the exercise until your calf muscles start to feel some exhaustion. Then stop to rest. That is one set. The capacity for the calves to perform isolated strength training like this varies greatly from person to person. For you, this may range from 5 repetitions up to 35. Or more. Just complete one set for starters. After a few times through the exercise, add a second set.

Just do the standard calf raise from a flat surface, and lower. There's no need to stand on a step and lower your heel below the level of the step; that is actually risky for the injured Achilles tendon. Stay with the flat surface for no risk and lots of effectiveness.

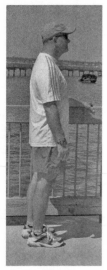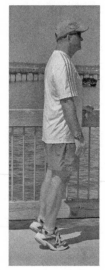

Figure 10: Standing calf raise starting position (left picture) and flexed position (right picture)

Once you build up adequate strength, you can perform the exercise while holding a pair of dumbbells to provide greater resistance. Or, just do more repetitions. Either way builds both strength and endurance; a routine with more weight and less repetitions sides toward strength building, less weight with more repetitions emphasizes endurance. Both are beneficial.

Walking Calf Raise

This is another simple yet effective exercise for strengthening those calf and soleus muscles; and it has kind of a lighthearted feel to it, I think. Want to hear simple? Here goes.

Just walk around the immediate area, and push yourself way up on your toes with each step. That's it. Up and down, up and down. Feels fun perhaps, but it's an effective strength and stability workout.

Take about 15 or 20 steps with each leg at first to get the hang of it. Work up to 70 to 100 after the first four or five sessions. You can do this by time instead, taking steps for maybe 20 seconds or so, then working up to over one minute eventually. 90 seconds is an ideal goal. Do this routine only every other day, to let your calf muscles get some rest on the off days.

Seated Reach-and-Pull Calf Flexion

This is a motion I've used with good results – and as far as I know, I thought it up! The Seated Reach-and-Pull is an isometric exercise, meaning you are working your muscle against an immovable object. In this case, that immovable object will be the floor. Any normal surface should work fine, be it carpet, vinyl, or a gym floor.

It doesn't matter if you are in stockings, shoes, or barefoot to do this exercise. It's done while seated, and a bench, chair or couch work as well as anything.

To begin, just reach your leg out (see Figure 11). Place the ball of your foot firmly on the floor, then lift your heel up a couple of inches. Start to pull that leg back, but as you do it, hook onto the floor with the ball of your foot and your toes. Grip hard with your foot, and attempt to drag that section of the floor to you (if the floor was well-made, it shouldn't budge!). Flex like this for a moment, between three to eight seconds or so, then rest. Repeat once more, then you're done with that leg. Perform it with your opposite leg as well. You might want to grip the chair with your hands so you don't pull yourself off the seat.

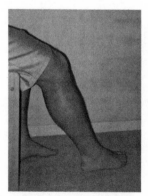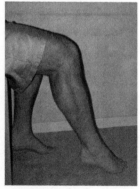

Figure 11: Seated Reach-and-Pull calf flexion starting position (left picture) and flexed position (right picture)

Do this every other day. After three or four of these Reach-and-Pull mini-workouts, add another flexion or two, each for just a few seconds of intense, strength-building tension.

This is a safe, non-impact, readily available exercise, and being an isometric resistance motion, it's capable of developing strength and stability like few other movements can. And it may be one of the best possible strengtheners you can do if your injury is acute and you can barely tolerate walking or standing. The isolated flexion of the Reach-and-Pull may still be possible despite the difficulty of other activities. It's therefore a great stability motion to rely upon and help ward off Achilles soreness, and keep it from returning once it disappears.

Resisted Calf Flexion

For this exercise you'll be seated, and you'll use either a towel or a pair of resistance bands if you have a pair.

Use both hands to hold the towel or resistance bands. Sit with your legs straightened in front of you, and wrap the middle section of the towel or the resistance bands around the balls of your feet (see Figure 12). Gently press your feet away from yourself until you're pointing your toes. At the same time, provide resistance with the strength of your arms and shoulders by pulling the towel or resistance bands towards yourself. The strength of your pull dictates how hard your calf muscles have to work. Hold at the extended position with a nice firm flexion, maintaining this position between three to eight seconds. Return to the starting position, and repeat once more.

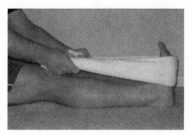 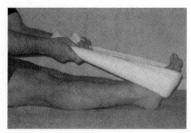

Figure 12: Resisted calf flexion starting position (left picture) and flexed position (right picture)

Do this flexion every other day, and you're sure to make strength and stability gains in the calf area. Much more resistance to Achilles tendinitis will be the result.

Crossover Stepping

In this simple and gentle exercise, you will be stepping out and doing a little locomotion. Kind of like a dance step. It can be done barefoot or with shoes on, it doesn't matter.

Specifically, you'll move sideways in one direction, then switch directions and go back the other way. To start:

Stand with your feet about shoulder width apart, then step your right foot across and in front of your left (see Figure 13). Moving in the same direction, bring the left foot over and place it next to the right, in the position from which you started. Then step the right foot again, this time behind the left. Move the left foot over and you'll be back to the starting position. Do this a few more times (unless you run out of room!), then reverse directions.

This low-intensity movement is ideal for gradual strengthening of all lower leg and foot muscles that associate with your Achilles tendon area. It will bring increased blood flow to the region, which the Achilles tendon can really use during its healing phase.

Perform this exercise every other day. If intense soreness occurs right away, stop at that point. Don't push past the pain. You'll improve over time. If there's no pain to speak of, do the Crossover Stepping motion for a minute or two at first. After you've done it a couple of times, work up to three minutes, then eventually get a good four or five minute workout with the Crossover Stepping exercise.

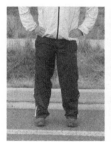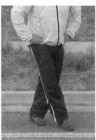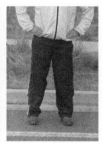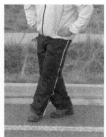

Figure 13: Crossover stepping series

***

So there you have it. Among the many calf-strengtheners you can do in the exercise universe, those six motions should encourage thorough reinforcement of the protective muscles that support your Achilles. These are not complicated exercises, nor are they very exciting. But they get the job done. It's pretty much a matter of buckling down and grinding out the repetitions.

After completing your session of any of these strengtheners, it is also a great time to do the stretching exercises. Your muscles will be warmed up, and having worked them you'll want to stretch them so as to prevent any cramping or tightening of the muscle tissues. We want to keep our muscles flexible.

Remember, strength training takes a while to adapt to. You may get sore a day or two after the first couple of times you specifically work out your calves. So don't overdo it, but at the same time, don't worry too much if a little soreness does occur. Of all the muscles in the body, the calves are some of the most resilient. They are used pretty much every day if a person walks at all, and are thus designed for plenty of rigor. So you can work them hard and with regularity, every other day or so being ideal. Do this and your calf muscles will serve as a better support system for your recuperating Achilles.

Keep Moving: Bike for Exercise

You may find yourself in a quandary regarding exercise due to your Achilles tendinitis ordeal. Perhaps you were in the good habit of walking for exercise, and that routine has now been tripped up by your foot injury. You struggle to walk around the kitchen, much less around the park. Even walking on a treadmill might hurt, despite its built-in cushion. Or if you like to hike, this reality of tenderness is even more true, given the steep nature and unpredictable texture of many trails.

And if you are in the acute stage of Achilles tendinitis, subjected to frequent stabs of pain nipping in your heel region, let's not even mention running. The pounding down of your bodyweight, coupled with the sheer number of footfalls realized on an average run, translates into a taxing experience for your injury. Yet you still want to keep moving, stay strong, and burn some calories. You may return to walking, hiking, and yes, even running in due time. But for now you need an alternative aerobic exercise source. What to do?

Consider biking.

Biking is a great cardiovascular workout. It is a non-weight bearing exercise, so stress and jarring on your Achilles area will be minimal. In addition, biking will provide incredible quadriceps conditioning. Your hamstrings, buttocks, hips, and calves will get in on the action too. It will help you improve endurance and strength, and add to the muscle mass in your legs and lower body. And with any gain in solid body mass, you will burn more energy even while resting. This quiet sizzle of calories will help you avoid any increase in body fat; it may even help you lose some. And any weight you can shed will mean that much less force on your feet, helping to speed your recovery.

You can ride a bike with intensity, but for moderate aerobic and strength training, feel free to ride casually. You'll still get plenty of exercise. As a matter of fact, once you slow way down, the resistance experienced to get back up to speed will be greater than if you were going fast, since you've lost forward momentum. The aerobic training and strength development will be substantial, and so will the energy you burn for weight control.

To protect your body, observe a couple of technique tips when biking. Make sure your knees go pretty much straight up and down;

don't angle them outwards, away from the bike. The straight up and down motion will exert less strain on your lower legs as well as your knees. Also, push the pedals with the middle of the foot, not the ball of the foot. The mechanics of pushing with the ball of the foot will stress the Achilles tendon. Pumping the pedals with the midfoot, on the other hand, will exert little strain there.

Of course, any benefits realized by riding a bike with wheels can also be attained by riding a stationary bike. In most ways, your body won't know the difference. Jump on either type of bike and move those pedals. You'll build endurance and some key leg muscles while you fry up lots of calories at the same time.

Keep Moving: Walk – Gently – for Exercise

To keep active, relieve stress, burn calories, and hasten your foot recovery, do some walking. Walking is a readily available, versatile, convenient, and inexpensive activity. It gives some folks peace of mind and as a result helps them improve their mood, stay positive, and even sleep better. And for such a seemingly gentle endeavor, it's quite effective in delivering results in terms of a workout.

If you are a runner, this chapter could be titled "Walk Instead of Run for Exercise." While in Achilles tendinitis recovery mode, you may want to avoid the high impact of running, and walk instead. Or at least consider replacing running with walking in the most acute phase of your injury. If you are not very active, but possibly acquired Achilles tendinitis by standing on your feet for very long periods of time, this may be a call for you to get more active and invigorate the muscles of your lower leg, ankle, and foot. Walking can greatly assist in some serious conditioning and strengthening of those areas, while subjecting you to very little impact.

The lack of impact realized while walking can be a huge plus. While walking, the force exerted upon your feet is only about one and a half times your body weight. While running, by comparison, your feet often endure up to ten times this amount.

The payoff in terms of calorie burn and conditioning gained while walking fast are undeniable, but you don't have to speed walk or race walk. In fact, when you walk slowly, momentum doesn't continue to carry you forward as it does when you walk very fast, so your muscles work a bit more to lift and propel you from a near dead stop. In truth, slow, medium, and brisk walking speeds will all provide a good workout. Walk at the speed with which you're most comfortable. And if you ever find yourself becoming out of breath, slow down. You just don't have to push yourself that hard to reap the benefits of walking.

Despite the low level of impact, you'll still want to walk in good form and with a normal foot strike. It can be tempting when suffering from Achilles tendinitis to limp or favor one side over the other. Resist making this mistake. Especially, be sure to avoid walking on the outside of the foot. This foot position may seem to give the injured area a rest, but in fact creates significant strain on the Achilles tendon, in particular at the point where it attaches to the heel bone.

To make matters worse, portions of your foot may then suffer injury, increasing your recovery dilemma.

Even though walking is relatively easy on your Achilles area, increase the distance you walk gradually. You may feel gung ho about your walking program, ready to exceed past distances, explore new places, and burn even more calories. This type of enthusiasm is a great thing, but use common sense at the same time. Walking will not stress your Achilles area like running, rugged hiking, or the fast stops and starts experienced in many sports. But it is still serious exercise. Walking will tax your muscles and connective tissue, which is actually one reason it's beneficial to you. But it can be overdone, especially when Achilles tendinitis is in its early stages. So if a given distance results in increased pain, versus simple muscle soreness, cut back on the length of your walk for the time being. If your injury is in the acute stage, where pain is quite sharp first thing in the morning, you can inflict upon your vulnerable lower legs additional damage by trying too much too soon. Resist that urge.

So if you read or hear something to the effect that a person should walk at least six days a week for thirty or forty minutes at a time minimum, take the advice with a grain of salt. You may or may not be ready for that type of exertion. Be enthused but cautious. Use a gradual approach. You'll work up to greater frequency and distance with time. I've read the suggested amount of 10% by which to increase your distance per week, but that's just a ballpark figure. You can lengthen your walks by even less than that each week and still make good progress. Or, if you find a walk location or routine you really like, don't feel pressure to increase the distance at all. Regular and consistent walks are far more important than long ones. That should be your priority for a walking program, not setting new records each week.

If you can only walk five or eight minutes at a time, due to time constraints or your level of injury, try to repeat these time increments a few times a day. The positive effects of walking can be realized in a cumulative sense. Five walking outings of five minutes each is roughly as beneficial as a contiguous twenty-five minute session. If short walks are all you can fit in to your day, take heart and keep at it.

To minimize any additional trauma your lower legs might experience as you make strides to get back in the game, see the "Maintain Low Impact Form" commentary in the "Protect and

Defend" section in Phase 1. Remember, Achilles tendinitis recovery is a tricky business. You need to keep moving, but avoid doing too much at the same time. And just as importantly, make sure you walk in good, supportive shoes, covered earlier in greater detail.

With that said, make a conscious effort to walk more, and plan the outings according to the amount your recovering Achilles tendon will allow. It will strengthen and tone your entire lower body, including those crucial muscles of the lower leg and foot. It may also help you sleep better, lift your spirits, and encourage you to stay committed to your overall recovery program. Include some variety, challenge yourself slowly but surely, and enjoy yourself.

Keep Moving: Swim for Exercise

If you want an exercise that is easy on your Achilles, subjects you to no impact, strengthens your entire body, and burns calories like crazy, go swimming. If you haven't done much swimming in recent years, it may be the perfect answer for a change of pace and a needed fitness boost.

I certainly am no expert on swimming techniques or strokes. I cannot outline a swimming regimen for fitness, but I know from experience that even a very short session will intensely work out a person's muscles and cardiovascular system.

For a person who has not used it much for exercise, swimming involves intense fitness demands. Even if you are in good condition for activities like biking, walking, and running, a swim can tax your aerobic and anaerobic abilities like nothing else. Swimming is an activity all its own. And for such a high value strengthening and calorie-consuming activity, swimming is surprisingly easy on the joints.

Your Achilles should experience no ill effects from swimming. It actually should get a little rest, even though your system will be going through grueling workouts. Swimming = lots of exertion, zero impact.

If you don't know how to swim, or it's been a long time since you have, consider swimming lessons. This period of recuperation on which you have embarked can be a time to try new things, and swimming might be a good challenge to tackle. And while you learn, you'll build endurance and strength while shedding quite a few calories. Maybe it will turn into a life-long activity for you.

Closely related to swimming is *deep water running*, which simulates running on land while wearing a flotation device. I've not yet tried this, but many athletes and coaches swear by it as a method of cross-training and injury recovery. Consider looking into a deep water running class at a local university or community pool. It could serve you well as a workout and an alternative to swimming if you're looking to mix up your activities further. And like swimming, your feet and lower legs will suffer no impact whatsoever.

For a total body workout that spares your Achilles injury of any abuse, dive into the swimming routine and get some serious exercise.

Phase 3:
Nurture

Create the best possible healing atmosphere that you can for your injury. Your body wants to heal; help it along.

Stay Well-Hydrated

Hydration is often overlooked as a major factor in injury recovery. But replenishing your body with plenty of water and other nutritious fluids will give your Achilles tendinitis recuperation a boost. Staying well-hydrated is very important to your overall health; if you're chronically dehydrated, Achilles tendinitis may represent just one of your worries.

Maintaining ideal hydration benefits your digestion, skin, hair, brain function, strength, and endurance. Adequate hydration will help ward off colds and flu. It will assist in heart health. If a person's hydration level drops even 5%, metabolism can slow as much as 30%. So any weight maintenance or weight loss efforts will be far easier with regular water intake (which in turn will help you heal from Achilles tendinitis: lower body weight = less Achilles tendon strain).

When you become dehydrated, so do your ligaments, muscles, and tendons. Connective tissue in the human body depends on water for elasticity and stability. Muscle function, including that of your calf and foot muscles, will be diminished with dehydration. This is exacerbated as your body's blood volume is reduced, or in other words the oxygen reaching the muscles becomes limited. Muscle performance will further suffer. This means weakening, tightness, and possible cramping. More strain on your Achilles tendon will result.

So make a conscious effort to consume plenty of fluids each day. And drink before you get thirsty. Under normal circumstances, with normal food intake, that fluid can be primarily water. Drink about 5-8 glasses of water a day. The water content in liquids like milk, orange juice, hot cocoa, and vegetable juice does count. Water contained in alcohol and in caffeinated drinks like cola and coffee do not, due to the diuretic effect these beverages have on the body.

Of course, it's best to do all things in moderation. When replacing lost fluids, there is no need to drink a gallon of water in a sitting. Try to rehydrate with the approximate amount of water you lost over time whether through normal activities or through vigorous work or exercise. If you are exercising heavily or enduring hot weather, in either case sweating profusely, you may want to consume a commercial sport drink to replace potassium, sodium, and other electrolytes at the same time that you rehydrate. This option is more effective for rejuvenation than plain water when fluid loss has been great, as described above. And it will help you avoid a condition known as hyponatremia, defined by a dangerously low concentration of sodium in the blood.

Hyponatremia results when heavy water loss takes place, and the only replacement you take for it is water alone; especially a large amount of water, which can cause the level of bloodstream minerals to drop. When mineral levels in your blood are low, such as sodium, water in your bloodstream may move into your brain, where concentrations of sodium are higher. This process is the normal attempt of human physiology to even things out. In this case, however, it can be bad news. The pressure in your brain could increase, and at the very least cause dizziness. It can also cause twitches, stupor, seizures, unconsciousness, and brain damage. So use good judgment when drinking back lost liquids.

Don't worry, an extra glass of water will not do this. A few extra glasses of plain water consumed at once might though, if you're dehydrated. When seeking replenishment, include some nutritious foods along with water, especially those containing potassium and sodium. Or as mentioned, consume a commercial sport drink, which will be designed to replace the lost minerals.

In short, be sensible when rehydrating. But by all means, make sure you take the time and effort to do it. Plan ahead and have drinks on hand before, during and after exercise, workdays, and outings of any kind. Adequate hydration can serve as a substantial aid in your healing process.

Massage Your Achilles Area

Consider using self-massage to accelerate your Achilles healing process. It involves a gentle palpitation of the area.

Do this carefully. You may be tempted to really dig your thumbs in, but go easy. Remember, there's not an evil life form in there that you are trying to crush; you're kneading the tissues of your injured Achilles heel region. Therefore, a light touch is the order of the day. Very forceful pressure could worsen the condition, as the area is already inflamed.

Proponents of massage believe that it encourages healing by manipulating the tissue at hand, and in so doing promotes relaxation, better blood flow, and the elimination of waste products. And in the case of Achilles tendinitis, massage can serve to break up scar tissue that is forming and allow the injured tissue to heal faster.

The actual technique for self-massaging your Achilles area is simple. Sit on the floor or a couch, bend your injured leg and bring that foot near you; then cup both hands around the front of your lower leg, right by the ankle. Place both thumbs upon your Achilles tendon, just above your heel bone and just below your calf, and begin the massage. Simply push in a few times, then run the thumbs up and down the length of the tendon. This serves to break up scar tissue and expedite healing. Apply slight pressure only. You can also cross one ankle over the opposite knee, and grasp the Achilles region with your thumb on one side of it and the fingers of that same hand on the other. Exert gentle pressure and kneading in the same way as you would with your thumbs.

Do this for a couple of minutes, and feel the result. If certain spots trigger sharp pain, discontinue the massage in that location, at least for the time being. You may benefit from the same action in the future, maybe in a few weeks once your healing has progressed. Or perhaps massage is not the best thing for your particular condition. You might have to experiment while being cautious.

You may, on the other hand, experience significant relief immediately. You'll have to feel the situation out, no pun intended. If gentle massage does give you immediate relief, do it regularly as part of your regimen. Once a day is not too often. This convenient procedure may do the trick to erase soreness, clear out waste products in the tissues of your Achilles area, and quicken your recovery. It may also diminish the return of pain as you resume activity. And, hey, sometimes it just feels good!

Massage Your Calf Muscles

Just as flexible, pliable calf muscles reduce the tension on the Achilles tendon, relaxed ones will have the same effect. You can ease the tension and help this set of muscles relax with massage. Feel free to massage your calf muscles with more vigor than you did your tendon. Within the realm of Achilles tendinitis, these muscles are not injured. So a bit more force can be put to work here without harm. Other than that, the procedure for this self-massage is similar to that used for the tendon. Sections of muscle where you feel soreness from working on your feet or exercising will be obvious, but massage the whole area, from the larger top section of the calf down to just above the heel area. The more the entire calf area is relieved of tightness and soreness, the less strain that your Achilles will undergo.

An additional benefit you will reap from a calf massage routine is the accelerated removal of waste products from the tissues, thereby gaining quicker recovery from any strength training or exercise you may have performed. You'll get stronger calf muscles in less time; strength gained in the calf area is always a boon to the solid foundation needed to recover from Achilles tendinitis, as well as ward off its return. So dig in.

Roll with It

With an ice-filled plastic bottle, that is. Take a bottle typical of the kind sport drinks and bottled water are sold in; a 16-ounce or 20-ounce size will do nicely. Fill it about ¾ full of tap water and freeze it.

Once the bottle is frozen solid and ready, sit on the floor, and place the bottle on the floor in front of you. For comfort, you might want to place a piece of cloth between your skin and the icy bottle. Then gently roll it back and forth underneath the length of your calf and Achilles tendon area. As you do it, you may maneuver your leg over the bottle as much as the bottle moves back and forth. It's an active massage method, actually a small workout in and of itself.

This is yet another way to massage your injured area, with a slightly different approach than a massage by hand. Like massaging your lower leg by hand, rolling the heel atop the bottle breaks up adhesions that may be forming on the traumatized tissue, and allows a more complete and rapid healing process to take place. Blood flow will be improved as well, which is in short supply in the Achilles area in all cases. The process will help to reduce inflammation as well as whisk away waste materials, further assisting your injury in a quicker repair.

When rolling your ailing leg atop an ice bottle, you're doing double duty for it: a stimulating massage coupled with an ice treatment. Take it easy in terms of pressure applied with an ice bottle, as it's pretty solid, and your living flesh isn't. Don't press too hard and make your already injured heel tissue more so.

You don't want to ice an injury to excess, so limit ice to 10 to 15 minutes a day at the most. If you have not yet iced your Achilles area on a given day, keep the ice bottle option in mind for quick relief. It fulfills ice and massage therapy at the same time.

Tighten Your Shoes

Supportive, well-fitting shoes can only do their job if the material of which they are composed fits the contours of your foot. Just as you should not wear shoes that are too big, you are better off if you don't leave shoes, even those with a proper fit, too loose on your feet. It may seem that since Achilles tendinitis has set in and you are battling the resulting inflammation, the looser the footwear the better. On the contrary: loose shoes can immensely irritate your injury. I found this through trial and error. At times, soreness would return unexpectedly when walking. I couldn't believe the difference it made when I tied any of the shoes I wore just a little tighter. Often the soreness creeping up in my heel would be reduced, and other times it would disappear completely.

Think snug here, not constricting. Certainly don't crank down and form a tourniquet with your laces. You just want each shoe to hug your foot a bit and not slide all over with each step. You may need to do some experimentation. At times, you might secure the laces too tight, and have to readjust them after a few steps. And if you are on a lengthy walk or standing for a long time, your feet may normally and naturally swell a little. This could also require an adjustment in your shoes' tightness. It might seem like a bother having to fiddle over and over with your shoes, but once you get them secured just right you'll see what I mean. The shape and construction of the shoes are then allowed to support your arch, cushion your landing, and control the motion of your feet. You'll find yourself stepping along easier and with less discomfort.

If you stop to rest, or you're going to be sitting for a while, by all means loosen the shoes for that period of time. Blood flow and relaxation will be at their optimum when shoes are loose. Let your circulation work in the best environment possible. The Achilles tendon area already has limited blood flow under the best conditions, so do what you can to help it along. Tighten the shoes back down when you get back up to walk, though. Sound like too much trouble? It can get annoying…but, this is your body we're talking about here. It's all part of the adjustments you make when recovering from Achilles tendinitis. Go to the extra trouble to snug your shoes to their optimum fit, and let them protect your feet and lower legs in the manner for which they were designed.

Elevate Your Lower Legs

Any chance you get to elevate your lower legs, do so. Elevating them will enhance blood flow and aid in the removal of waste products from the injury. Elevation reduces the blood pressure in the area and thus the swelling. Additionally, the improved circulation will allow better delivery of nutrients to the injured tissue, helping the tissue heal. Your recovery process will speed up as a result.

You basically want to elevate your lower legs above the level of your heart. Nothing too scientific here. The most practical way to do this is to simply lie on your back and prop your feet up. You can use a couple of pillows, or maybe even the couch or a cushioned chair.

Try to elevate the lower legs for 8-15 minutes. If you can only fit in 5 minutes or so at a given time, still treat yourself to it. Elevation of the lower legs is a course of action where you can feel the relief immediately. Especially if you've just been on your feet for a long time or you've been out walking or running. Once you do it a time or two, you'll probably need no further encouragement. Your Achilles area will feel noticeable relief. Not to mention, the session might give you a chance to unwind, read, or rest, so the benefits of powering down to prop up your lower legs may be multiple.

Whoever thought doing so little could do so much? Keep this effortless tactic in mind and use it to encourage your progress back to healthier feet and heels. All while you lie down, stretch out, and relax.

Get Enough Sleep

Spend a little more time in bed and you might heal more quickly as a result. To expedite your recuperation from Achilles tendinitis, it's in your interest to get plenty of sleep. It seems counterintuitive, but here's why it works.

During sleep your body takes many measures to restore itself; among these processes is the generation of Human Growth Hormone, a healing hormone your system naturally produces. During deep sleep, your body creates higher amounts of it.

In addition to helping you repair injuries, Human Growth Hormone enhances a slow, steady calorie burn; this helps regulate body fat and prevent excess weight gain in case you're forced to become inactive. Along the same line, Human Growth Hormone regulates your body's sensitive chemical balance, which helps control your appetite. So with no extra effort on your part, getting a good night's sleep allows you to manage your weight; sleep's weight control abilities can compensate for the fewer calories you may burn due your being laid up.

Researchers have found that significant changes in the levels of the hormones ghrelin and leptin occur when you get less than 5 hours of sleep. After a few consecutive nights of poor sleep you may find yourself with an out-of-control appetite; this is mostly because sleep deprivation increases ghrelin and decreases leptin below normal levels. This sensitive hormone balance helps control your appetite. Ghrelin is used to whet your appetite; if its level is excessive, your appetite will be excessive as well.

Weight control and injury recovery aside, do you want to live sleep-deprived anyway? The inability to sleep can be a medical issue, and much more complex than we can completely discuss here. But many situations of sleep deprivation are caused by individual choices, like staying up late to surf the web, play video games, or, amazingly, watch late night TV programs even when sleepy. (Could these shows possibly be worth losing sleep over?)

Enough with my soap box moment. Here are some tips to acquire restorative sleep:

    – Avoid caffeine a few hours before you plan to sleep. Old advice but still worth mentioning. Caffeine consumed eight or nine hours before you sleep will usually be cleared from your system before bedtime; caffeine consumed an hour or two before that time usually won't be.

– If you drink alcohol, pay attention to how it affects you and your sleeping experience. If you need to cut back, you'll know it. Then do it.

– If deep, sound sleep eludes you, keep in mind that lying still, in a neutral relaxed state, provides many of the same benefits as deep sleep. It can make for a long night just lying there waiting for sleep, but try to stay calm and simply rest. Above all, don't let anxiety about not sleeping ironically cause you to not sleep. Knowing the fact that calm rest is a close second to deep sleep can, interestingly enough, help you transition into sound sleep. That's been my experience.

– Read a book, paper, or magazine an hour or so before retiring, in place of using a computer or watching TV. The electronic media are believed to disturb normal sleep, in some cases and for some reason, whereas reading from print materials actually encourages preparation for sleep.

– If you get a chance to take a nap, do it. Not many of us have time for naps in today's sometimes-crazy world, but go for it if the opportunity arises.

    This thought has not been without controversy. In recent decades a few "experts" have proclaimed that naps are useless, and that they disrupt nighttime sleep. And, of all things, that they age you. Balderdash. If we weren't meant to take naps, and if the body and brain didn't yearn for them, we wouldn't take them. Treat yourself to a nap when you can. It will encourage injury recovery.

– Go to sleep a little earlier if you can. Early birds wake up refreshed and seize the day, while night owls are the ones still walking around in a near zombie state at 9:00 AM, babbling about not being a morning person. For best results on your injury recuperation endeavor, you have to do what's best for your body and brain. Adequate sleep will be a big help in your recovery efforts. If for you that means going to sleep a little earlier, choose that option.

I believe this is a rare time that you'll see a firm recommendation to make sleep a priority for wound healing. Like adequate hydration, the need for a good night's sleep is often undervalued and overlooked when it comes to recovery from bodily injuries. For wound healing, trust me…better yet, trust science: adequate sleep can make a difference.

Consume Plenty of Antioxidants

To keep your body's healing powers on overdrive, fortify yourself with a regular dose of antioxidants. Your body already helps protect itself by producing certain enzymes that serve as antioxidants. You can add to this protection by consuming antioxidant-rich foods.

What purpose do antioxidants serve?

The physiological process of oxidation occurs normally as part of your body's functioning, such as in respiration and metabolism. However, oxidation also produces the deleterious byproducts known as "free radical" molecules. The incidence of physical exertion, injury, and stress will increase the normal quantity of free radicals, and they will then accumulate more quickly. If their presence becomes too great, they can cause cell damage, which is part of the "oxidative stress" process. This process can bring about several negative consequences, among which is the slowing of your body's ability to heal.

Perhaps the most dramatic benefit of antioxidants in your diet is their conquest over oxidants, i.e., free radicals. Antioxidants detect and scavenge these unwanted free radicals. The free radicals are then neutralized and eliminated.

As a consequence, antioxidants reduce inflammation, which improves circulation. Tissue damage will be minimized; damaged tissue will be more quickly repaired. And healing will be thus accelerated. In a similar fashion, you will recover from workouts and strengthening exercises more easily. So you'll become stronger that much faster.

As a nice side benefit, those foods which contain lots of antioxidants also tend to be highly nutritious. Mind and body will function better in every way when your nutrition level is tip-top. You'll feel fully operational with fewer calories when you supply yourself with high-nutrient fuel. What's more, antioxidants allow your system to better utilize nutrients you've consumed. You'll get more "bang for the bite" from the food components you eat.

How can you make sure your normal diet includes enough antioxidants? To simplify matters, if you regularly eat fruits and vegetables, you will get at least a fair supply of antioxidants. So make sure you do. To really boost your system's recuperative abilities, check out the following list of antioxidant top performers. Include some or all of them as part of your regular eating routine.

Excellent antioxidant sources:
Blueberries, strawberries, cherries, apples, grapes, cranberries, raspberries, blackberries, vegetable oils, olives, seeds, peanuts, walnuts, almonds, avocado, whole wheat, beans, broccoli, seafood, beef, pork, chicken, brown rice, cantaloupe, peppers, spinach, squash, sweet potatoes, and citrus fruit.

In addition, black and green teas are loaded with antioxidants; so if you already enjoy either of these, continue drinking them. And good news for coffee drinkers: recent studies have found coffee, both regular and decaf, to be loaded with antioxidants. Yay!

Some other interesting antioxidant sources are red wine, dark chocolate, and honey. This does not mean you should gobble down a whole chocolate bar, eat a jar of honey, and wash it down with an entire bottle of wine. Moderation in all things. Think sips and morsels when it comes to these very sweet items.

You'll want to partake of antioxidant-rich foods as part of your Achilles tendinitis recovery process, to be sure. But really, eating such foods is a good habit to get into for life. Your injury will heal quicker, but also, a high antioxidant intake will help ward off illness and just plain make you feel better. Get into the routine of consuming food which contains plenty of antioxidants, and your injury recovery program and overall health will take a big step forward.

Track Your Food Intake

There is no getting around it: a lower body weight will mean less strain on your Achilles tendon. If you carry a little extra weight, and most of us do, now is the time to commit to reducing some of that excess. Just a few less pounds on your frame can result in significant relief to your injured heel region.

Reams of books have been written on weight loss. This book is not one of them. I will not turn this into a weight loss seminar, but at the same time, I'd be derelict in my duties if I failed to mention the subject of body weight while discussing Achilles tendinitis recovery. And I won't just blurt out "Lose weight." That would oversimplify a very complex issue. For many folks, weight control is a life-long challenge. And that includes me.

So I'll propose one course of action that you can try. It is the least original advice you may have ever heard. It's old advice. In fact, it's almost worn out advice. But it's the type of advice that, if followed, always pays off.

Write down each and every thing you eat in a given day.

Doesn't sound too profound or exciting, does it? But…when was the last time you did it? If you choose to follow this advice, I think you will find three things:

- You're probably eating more than you think.
- You're letting less-than-desirable foods sneak into your daily intake.
- You're able to eat plenty, actually indulge yourself, if you cut the diabolical but always available junk food from your diet.

And if your experience is anything like mine, you'll skip a lot of bad food choices when you're faced with writing each one down. Keep the recording of your intake basic for best results. You'll want an uncomplicated system in order to keep with it for a sustained time period. Not to mention, to start doing it in the first place. Perhaps use a pocket-sized calendar or even a post-it or two during the day. Then copy it down later into a log, using something as simple as a notebook or a tablet.

Find a nutrition book that lists calorie counts, or bookmark one of the numerous websites out there which contain the information. Then track the associated calories of each item. Don't have access to these resources, and don't know the calorie count on a given item? Guess at it. You can look it up later. The important thing is to list the item and help yourself become aware of what you are eating. (Of course, record what you drink each day also. Many calories can slip in quickly through beverages if you let them.)

Soon you'll get the system down and the calorie counts memorized. After the first few days, try to winnow down the calories slightly. Maybe reduce them 5% or so, 10% at the most. Change your eating habits slow but steady. Try this regimen for just two weeks. You may be surprised at what you find, and at the results you experience. If you like what you see, stick with it for another week or two.

Logging what you eat each day will not only help you monitor how much you take in, it will also help you track the *types* of calories you consume. This leads me to qualify the statement made above regarding bodyweight as it relates to Achilles tendinitis. A heavier body due to lots of muscle will in fact subject your Achilles tendon to a little more stress than a lighter body would. But keep the muscle. It's too important as a fat burner to lose it. Muscle on your frame boosts the quietly purring furnace of your metabolism a bit; you will burn extra calories just maintaining the muscle. Healthier food choices allow you to maintain the muscle that much easier. And, happily, lower your body fat percentage instead.

So, what exactly should you eat on a regular basis for best results? This is an enormous subject, but perhaps it's best to begin with what you should *not* eat. Extensive studies, journals, and textbooks have been completed on the subject of nutrition. But as for foods to avoid, you knew most of the answers back in grade school. Here are just a few obvious examples of items to limit or completely avoid: donuts, cheese puffs, pre-wrapped snack cakes, apple fritters, super-sized french fries, fast food hamburgers and hotdogs made with fiber-free white buns, most types of candy, and cream-filled long johns. Just to name a few.

Am I making your mouth water? Sorry. But I think you get the picture. And I bet you already knew the items mentioned were ill-advised. The stuff is tempting though, isn't it? And it's so readily available nowadays. To help you dig your heels in and resist temptations like these, write them down when you eat any of them.

You will find that when diligently tracking your intake, the notion of documenting a gooey snack item, which took you maybe two minutes total to eat, then jotting a whopping 400, 500, or 600 as the calorie value, will in fact be daunting. You will start to think twice about such transgressions if you hold yourself accountable in writing. Tracking your intake will help you form better eating habits.

What can you replace these questionable goodies with? I'm not a nutritionist, but after researching the subject for myself, I found some things that work for me. Here are my suggestions.

Fruits and vegetables should represent a mainstay in your diet. No surprise there. But once you wean yourself off sweet snacks filled with refined sugar, you might not believe how sweet and satisfying a piece of fruit tastes. Try it for a while. Barring any allergies to them, include a variety of nuts in your diet. Not only are nuts convenient snacks, but they contain large amounts of protein and heart-healthy fats. Replace white bread, noodles, and rice with piles of veggies at dinner now and then. You'll get full sooner and stay satisfied much longer.

Avoid any product that contains hydrogenated oils, also called "trans fats." Trans fats are oils artificially processed for longer storage; they are unnatural, of little food value, and hard on your cardiovascular system. For good sources of fats, turn to oils such as coconut, flaxseed, and olive oils. Like nuts, they contain the kind of healthy fats you want in your diet.

Meats are good in moderation. This may be up for debate, but many traditional food gurus insist any naturally occurring fat is pretty good for you, and will nourish you and satiate you for hours. In any case, a given amount of calories from fat will *always* fill you for a longer period than the same amount from a processed carbohydrate source.

Avoid too much corn oil and safflower oil, as they are too high in Omega-6 fats; you need more Omega-3 fats actually, to balance the out-of-whack proportion of Omega-3 to Omega-6 fats resulting from heavy processing by the food industry. So eat fish, from freshwater or the ocean, on a regular basis. Fish are low in calories, packed with protein, and certain types, especially sardines, mackerel, trout, and wild salmon, serve as a source of healthful Omega-3 fats. Walnuts are another great source of Omega-3 fats.

For a sweetener, it's hard to beat honey. Honey digests slower than table sugar, so you avoid the quick surge and crash often associated with sweet foods. Honey contains antioxidants, and is sweet enough to satisfy those desperate cravings a person gets from time to time. Mix a tablespoon of honey with a dash of cinnamon, and you have a tiny but powerfully sweet and healthy treat.

If you long for candy, and can't hold back, hit the chocolate. Choose dark chocolate if it's available. It too contains antioxidants. And the intense flavor of dark chocolate should stop a sweet tooth in its tracks. Chocolate has lots of calories though, so limit the portions you imbibe in.

Don't obsess over losing weight. Track your food intake, keep exercising, and see where you can substitute better foods for the high-calorie, low-value ones. Whatever happens, happens. Even if you don't lose an ounce, your system will be fortified with higher quality nutrients with which to repair your injured Achilles.

Tracking your food intake daily almost guarantees you'll eat a little less, and the foods you do eat will be healthier. And you may painlessly lose some weight in the process.

Phase 4:
Bolster Your Spirit to Accelerate Healing

Just as physical progress is crucial to your recovery, so is the can-do **attitude** that will keep you on track and feed the flames of success.

Avoid Jumping Back in Too Soon

Recovery from a bout with Achilles tendinitis is quite the balancing act, isn't it? You must strategically restrain yourself from harmful activities, giving yourself a break from the source of your injury. Yet, experts generally agree that exercise and strengthening are not only OK but required for recovery. So far you've been encouraged to stretch, strengthen, move, and eat better. After all that, you must feel ready to get back into the action, maybe with even more vigor than before.

Not so fast. In addition to all its other annoying aspects, Achilles tendinitis has a nasty habit of recurring. So proceed with caution.

This advice might sound like lecturing, but it can't hurt to receive a reminder. Persevering on a recuperation or prevention plan is where commitment comes into play. And commitment is crucial to overcome Achilles tendinitis. Sometimes it entails gung ho enthusiasm for new strengthening exercises and stretches, active rehab, things you can do with vigor. But sometimes it means denial. Sometimes it means backing off. Sometimes it's boring. It's difficult to resist the temptation to jump back in too soon. But to speed healing and avoid reinjury, you have to surrender to the need for rest. If you do all other parts of the recovery plan faithfully but continue stressing your injury, you are possibly sabotaging yourself.

Remember: nurture your body, not your pride.

For instance, if you were able to make special arrangements at a job to accommodate your condition, see if you can transition back into your normal duties little by little. Don't declare full recovery too quickly. Work back into the groove slowly over time.

When it comes to walking for exercise, push yourself a little, but remember to rein yourself in at the same time. Especially if you feel really revved up, as in trying to break your old records by a long shot. Walking is low impact and therefore pretty ideal as a recovery activity, but it can be overdone just like anything else. Keep all things in moderation when you're recuperating.

If you are a runner, start back up with very conservative durations and speed. Forget what you used to do in terms of time and distance. When transitioning back into the "old you," you need to do it gradually. Be enthused, but don't erase your recent progress with extreme enthusiasm that turns out to be your undoing.

Maybe rearrange your goals from what they were previously. Don't think of this as setting your sights lower. Think of it as taking care of yourself. I'd say the fact that you can get back into running at all is its own victory. Same with resuming walking, hiking, and other sports you love. Have fun, but not too much fun!

And, it should be said, keep on with your recovery exercises. Continue to stretch every day. Do the strengthening exercises on a regular basis. More flexible and stronger soleus and calf muscles will only continue to help you. Make sure to eat good food and avoid unhealthy food. Don't eat huge quantities. Make these positive actions part of your daily routine.

Ease back into things. However humble your progress is at first, remember that you're making a comeback; enjoy the excitement and accomplishment that goes along with it.

Visualize Success and Move On

Since beginning your battle with Achilles tendinitis, how do you see yourself? As an invalid? As a cripple? Or as a bundle of strength and energy, stymied by a physical setback just for the moment? Do you picture never-ending misery from your pain, or success and pain-free Achilles tendons around the corner?

I believe the difference between a negative and a positive attitude, and thus the self image you maintain, can lead to very different results as you try to recuperate from Achilles tendinitis. A positive attitude can serve as a major factor in a speedy recovery process. Similarly, so too can your self-image.

The body and mind are unquestionably linked. Ever had a tension headache? Most people have. If and when you've had one, do you recall anyone clamping a big vice on your head and tightening it down? Or were you hit on the head with a rubber mallet just before the headache hit? Probably not. Most likely, the headache was caused by what you perceived about the events happening around you; events that were frustrating and helped you get stressed out. What went on in your mind led to a quite tangible physical result. Your mind and body can be very closely linked. Negative thoughts can have very real physical manifestations. So for optimum healing, be careful what you think about and dwell upon.

Experiments which involve the use of placebo medications often demonstrate good examples of the power of the human mind. A recent study at Columbia University tested the effect of belief as it relates to physical reactions and sensations. Participants were administered two instances of skin cream; one batch was said to reduce pain, the other to have no effect. The cream was placed on different parts of the subjects' arms, and heat was then applied to the point of causing a burning sensation. The subjects reported those spots covered with pain-reducing cream felt less pain compared to the areas covered with the neutral cream. Brain scans measuring pain response confirmed their reports.

The applied creams were exactly the same.

What you tell yourself and what you believe may materialize into reality.

During these trying times of injury recovery, it may be difficult to see the bright side of things, day in and day out. You may not always experience high levels of cheer, but be especially careful of letting pessimism consume you. A pessimistic outlook can promote a negative self-image, and among other things increase your level of stress. This undesirable combination can progress to the point where you may feel defeated, helpless, and hopeless in the struggle against your heel condition…which in turn can spawn panic. When you panic, you experience the dramatic "fight or flight" response. This response is your body's inborn reaction to real or imagined threats, one that prepares you to fight back or run away. You would never want to live without the ability to summon the fight or flight response; it can save your life in an emergency. But having it activated regularly for a long period of time can really wear on a person. And it can slow down your recuperation process.

For instance, a by-product of extreme stress such as that caused by the fight or flight response is the hormone cortisol. Among other things, the presence of high cortisol levels can stymie your body's immune response. Dr. Frank M. Perna, a psychologist and associate professor at Boston University, explained this in the New York Times. "Athletes who are training hard are breaking down muscle," he said, "and cortisol will impede the body's ability to repair muscles, making them more likely to get injured or exacerbate a chronic injury." In a similar way, the less cortisol and other nasty by-products of stress you have saturating your tissues, the better your progress will be when healing from Achilles tendinitis.

High stress also increases muscle tension, tightening those muscles up when they should be loose and flexible to help you move efficiently and protect you. Tense muscles are more susceptible to strains, tears, and cramps. And in your particular case, those key muscle groups of the lower leg and foot won't operate smoothly, and support for your vulnerable Achilles tendon will be minimized. Nobody can lead a completely stress-free existence, but do what you can to avoid stressful scenarios, and relieve stress in ways that work for you. Commit to it.

On a less scientific note, a nasty bout with Achilles tendinitis can bring on good old-fashioned discouragement. If you're feeling down and whipped as the condition endures, how likely are you to carry through with efforts needed to heal yourself of Achilles tendinitis? Not very. Of course, being optimistic and on top of your game is not always easy. It's tough to see everyone else walking and running all over without a hint of pain, while you can't walk around the block. Allowed to run rampant, this cloudy sky engulfing your spirit could change your way of living. You might get in the habit of sulking, become sedentary and lethargic, and lead a self-defeating existence. Self-pity, which serves no valuable purpose, could take the place of ambition and activity. Many people lead their whole life without acquiring a condition like Achilles tendinitis. Why you?

Well, why not you? People face all sorts of challenges, and Achilles tendinitis just happens to be one you're facing currently. The condition itself is impediment enough; you can't afford any extra negativity. Don't picture yourself as an invalid or a cripple. You're strong, resilient, and capable, but sidelined with a nasty and sadly very prevalent condition. But it's a temporary condition, if you choose to beat it. Whether you spend your present moments in a state of enthusiasm or a state of gloom, the time will go by either way. Decide to be positive, remember the situation won't be around forever, and count on each day being another step toward full recovery.

An important practice recommended to athletes by sports psychologists is the act of positive visualization. The basic concept involves picturing over and over a perfect performance, a flawless execution of the actions, and a successful outcome. The athlete is never to imagine tripping up, or missing a swing, or dropping a ball. Only success. Only the perfect outcome. And with these images of an ideal performance follows the realization of it. Many athletes swear by this visualization-to-reality process. In a similar way, you can picture a successful outcome to your ordeal. See in your mind's eye fully functional, pain-free lower legs. Even try to feel them. Know with certainty that your Achilles tendons can return to a stable, healthy state. And in a matter of time, they will. In the high-stakes game of Achilles tendinitis recovery, you now know what it takes to win. So carry through on this knowledge, and expect to win.

Don't forget to practice the proper caution and engage in sensible activities, but move on nonetheless. Once you've committed to your recovery plan and stuck with it a while, the routine will become second nature. As will the better choices and better habits. So don't proceed with your day in fear, proceed with confidence. If you go a little too far or do a little too much, ratchet your efforts back a bit. If you make your lower legs ache now and again by walking or standing more than you should have, know that you haven't canceled out all your good efforts. Your body is adaptable, and will help you overcome any indiscretions and slight reinjuries you may experience. Just learn from it and adjust.

Make peace with yourself that your Achilles tendinitis condition requires some significant rest, and avoidance of those factors that caused it in the first place. However inconvenient this is to you. Give your legs, heels, and feet a break and allow them a chance to heal. You'll be back in action that much sooner.

Achilles tendinitis is an obstacle, and a big one. But people overcome all kinds of obstacles. Don't dwell on the problem to excess. Make an unwavering commitment to help yourself heal. And while you're at it, keep living your life; adjust your lifestyle as needed to recuperate. Be confident and patient, do what needs to be done, and you *will* prevail against Achilles tendinitis.

Stretching and Strengthening Log

On the following couple of pages you'll find a convenient log to track your stretching and strengthening activities. Simply check off the stretches and strengthening moves as you perform them each day. You by no means need to perform every single move every day (see the appropriate sections for frequency recommendations); this log is simply meant as a way for you to keep track.

	Start date:							Date:						
	M	T	W	Th	F	S	Su	M	T	W	Th	F	S	Su
Calf stretch (Fig 3 or Fig 5)														
Seated calf stretch (Fig 4)														
Wall soleus stretch (Fig 6)														
Arch Plus stretch (Fig 7)														
Hamstring stretch (Fig 8)														
Seated calf raise (Fig 9)														
Standing calf raise (Fig 10)														
Walking calf raise														
Reach-and-Pull calf flexion (Fig 11)														
Resisted calf flexion (Fig 12)														
Crossover stepping (Fig 13)														

	Date:							Date:						
	M	T	W	Th	F	S	Su	M	T	W	Th	F	S	Su
Calf stretch (Fig 3 or Fig 5)														
Seated calf stretch (Fig 4)														
Wall soleus stretch (Fig 6)														
Arch Plus stretch (Fig 7)														
Hamstring stretch (Fig 8)														
Seated calf raise (Fig 9)														
Standing calf raise (Fig 10)														
Walking calf raise														
Reach-and-Pull calf flexion (Fig 11)														
Resisted calf flexion (Fig 12)														
Crossover stepping (Fig 13)														

	Date:							Date:						
	M	T	W	Th	F	S	Su	M	T	W	Th	F	S	Su
Calf stretch (Fig 3 or Fig 5)														
Seated calf stretch (Fig 4)														
Wall soleus stretch (Fig 6)														
Arch Plus stretch (Fig 7)														
Hamstring stretch (Fig 8)														
Seated calf raise (Fig 9)														
Standing calf raise (Fig 10)														
Walking calf raise														
Reach-and-Pull calf flexion (Fig 11)														
Resisted calf flexion (Fig 12)														
Crossover stepping (Fig 13)														

About the Author

Patrick Hafner has been involved in fitness and conditioning for over 30 years. He competed for 15 years in wrestling sports, winning numerous state, regional, and international titles, and has worked as a strength training adviser and judo instructor. As a hiking enthusiast, Patrick has explored trails all over North America and Europe. As a runner, he has completed over 80 races. Patrick holds a B.S. in Kinesiology from the University of Minnesota.

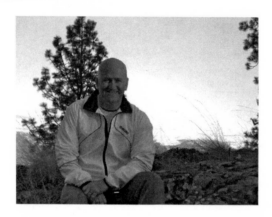